Down Syndrome

Down Syndrome

Neurobehavioural Specificity

Edited by

JEAN-ADOLPHE RONDAL

Unité de Psycholinguistique, Département des Sciences Cognitives, Université de Liège, Liège, Belgium
Facoltà delle Scienze della Formazione, Università degli Studi di Udine, Udine, Italy

and

JUAN PERERA

Centro Principe de Asturias, Universidad de las Islas Baleares, Palma de Mallorca, Baleares, Spain

John Wiley & Sons, Ltd

Other Wiley Editorial Offices

John Wiley & Sons Inc., 111 River Street, Hoboken, NJ 07030, USA

Jossey-Bass, 989 Market Street, San Francisco, CA 94103-1741, USA

Wiley-VCH Verlag GmbH, Boschstr. 12, D-69469 Weinheim, Germany

John Wiley & Sons Australia Ltd, 42 McDougall Street, Milton, Queensland 4064, Australia

John Wiley & Sons (Asia) Pte Ltd, 2 Clementi Loop #02-01, Jin Xing Distripark, Singapore
129809

John Wiley & Sons Canada Ltd, 6045 Freemont Blvd, Mississauga, ONT L5R

Wiley also publishes its books in a variety of electronic formats. Some content that appears
in print may not be available in electronic books.

Library of Congress Cataloging-in-Publication Data

Down syndrome : neurobehavioral specificity / edited by Jean-Adolphe
    Rondal & Juan Perera.
     p. cm.
    Includes bibliographical references and index.
    ISBN-13: 978-0-470-01948-1 (pbk. : alk. paper)
    ISBN-10: 0-470-01948-4 (pbk. : alk. paper)
    1. Down syndrome. 2. Mental retardation. 3. Neurogenetics.
    4. Behavior genetics. I. Rondal, J. A. II. Perera, Juan.
    [DNLM: 1. Down Syndrome. 2. Neurobehavioral Manifestations.
    3. Genetics, Behavioral. WS 107 D74895 2006]
    RJ506.D68D69 2006
    618.92′858842 – dc22

                        2006006498

A catalogue record for this book is available from the British Library
ISBN-13   978-0-470-01948-1
ISBN-10   0-470-01948-4

Typeset by SNP Best-set Typesetter Ltd., Hong Kong
Printed and bound in Great Britain by TJ International Ltd, Padstow, Cornwall

This book is printed on acid-free paper responsibly manufactured from sustainable forestry
in which at least two trees are planted for each one used for paper production.

Contents

Donna Spiker, Early Childhood Program, Center for Education and Human Services, SRI International, Menlo Park, California, USA

Mariusz Walus, Department of Developmental Neurobiology, Institute for Basic Research in Developmental Disabilities, New York, USA

Krystyna E. Wisniewski, Department of Developmental Neurobiology, Institute for Basic Research in Developmental Disabilities, New York, USA

Contents

Contributors

Giorgio Albertini, Child Development Department, IRCCS San Raffaele Pisana Hospital, Rome, Italy

Darlynne A. Devenny, Department of Psychology, Institute for Basic Research in Developmental Disabilities, New York, USA

Lea Ferrari, Dipartimento di Psicologia dello Sviluppo e della Socializzazione, Università degli Studi di Padova, Padova, Italy

Deborah J. Fidler, Human Development and Family Studies, College of Applied Human Sciences, Colorado State University, Fort Collins, Colorado, USA

Adam A. Golabek, Department of Developmental Neurobiology, Institute for Basic Research in Developmental Disabilities, New York, USA

Giovanni Maria Guazzo, Centro NeapoliSanit, Ottaviano (Napoli), Italy

Robert M. Hodapp, Department of Special Education, Vanderbilt University, Nashville, Tennessee, USA

Elizabeth Kida, Department of Developmental Neurobiology, Institute for Basic Research in Developmental Disabilities, New York, USA

Lynn Nadel, Department of Psychology, University of Arizona, Tucson, Arizona, USA

Laura Nota, Dipartimento di Psicologia dello Sviluppo e della Socializzazione, Università degli Studi di Padova, Padova, Italy

Sonia Palminiello, Child Development Department, IRCCS San Raffaele Pisana Hospital, Rome, Italy

David Patterson, Department of Biological Sciences, Eleanor Roosevelt Institute, University of Denver, Denver, Colorado, USA

Juan Perera, Centro Principe de Asturias, Universidad de las Islas Baleares, Palma de Mallorca, Baleares, Spain

Ausma Rabe, Department of Developmental Neurobiology, Institute for Basic Research in Developmental Disabilities, New York, USA

Alberto Rasore Quartino, Ospedale Galliera, Genova, Italy

Jean-Adolphe Rondal, Unité de Psycholinguistique, Département des Sciences Cognitives, Université de Liège, Liège, Belgium. Facoltà delle Scienze della Formazione, Università degli Studi di Udine, Udine, Italy

Salvatore Soresi, Dipartimento di Psicologia dello Sviluppo e della Socializzazione, Università degli Studi di Padova, Padova, Italy

Donna Spiker, Early Childhood Program, Center for Education and Human Services, SRI International, Menlo Park, California, USA

Mariusz Walus, Department of Developmental Neurobiology, Institute for Basic Research in Developmental Disabilities, New York, USA

Krystyna E. Wisniewski, Department of Developmental Neurobiology, Institute for Basic Research in Developmental Disabilities, New York, USA

Foreword

This book resulted from a research symposium organised by ASNIMO, the Mallorcan association for Down syndrome, sponsored by the Presidency of the Balearic Islands government and the University of the Balearic Islands. It took place in Palma de Mallorca, Spain, in the last days of February 2005. We are grateful to the fine group of distinguished colleagues who agreed to participate in the symposium and to expand their contributions into chapters suitable for international publication. The economic assistance of Gabriel Escarrer (Sol Melia Hotels and Resorts), Miguel Fluxá (Fundación Iberostar) and Mr Luis and Mrs Carmen Riu (Riu Hotels and Resorts) was essential for this symposium. We would also like to express our appreciation to Nicky Skinner, Emma Hatfield, Marc Weide, Anne Bassett, from Wiley, and David Michael, copy editor, for their help in collecting and integrating the chapters into book format. We are pleased to acknowledge the collaboration and dedicated attention of our assistants and secretaries, Carmen Crespo, Raquel Marin, Cinta Gonzales, Paola Spadaro, Anastasia Piat and Laurence Docquier in the preparation of the final manuscript.

Jean-Adolphe Rondal and Juan Perera

1 Specificity in Down Syndrome: A New Therapeutic Criterion

J. PERERA

Centro Príncipe de Asturias, Palma de Mallorca, Baleares, Spain

SUMMARY

Now that the human genome has been mapped, connections between genetic code and its ultimate effects on health, intelligence and behaviour are being made swiftly. Consequently, the study of 'specificity' is of great interest in the field of Down syndrome (DS).

Specificity

- allows us to understand DS not just in terms of its aetiology but also its consequences
- provides the foundation for more effective and direct intervention
- is the defining principle of specialised DS associations, which differ from those associations serving individuals with non-specific mental retardation

This introductory chapter will attempt to provide a broad picture of the subject, the various approaches to it (at the individual level and the systemic level), its methodology and the most interesting findings from the genetic, clinical, biomedical and practical perspectives.

We faced the challenge of trying to define and document, using scientific criteria and inter-syndrome comparisons, possible specificity among syndromes that include mental retardation (as is the case with DS). From the intervention perspective it would appear that the specific characteristics of a syndrome require specific methods whereas non-specific characteristics require more general methods, which can be extended to other syndromes. Hence the title of this chapter.

INTRODUCTION

What is specificity? How can one study it scientifically? What do we know today about specificity in DS? What practical consequences can be derived

Down Syndrome: Neurobehavioural Specificity. Edited by JA Rondal and J Perera.
© 2006 John Wiley & Sons Ltd.

from specificity with respect to more effective and direct intervention? These are some of the issues that are discussed in this chapter, which aims to introduce the difficult problem of specificity in DS and to give coherence to each of the following chapters.

Do individuals with DS possess specific attributes that characterise their development during the first stages of life – in their neuropsychological development, in their memory, in their intellectual function, in their learning, in their linguistic development, in their personality and behaviour, in their ageing or in their healthcare?

The scientific analysis of specificity in DS is today a subject of extraordinary interest and relevance for three reasons:

- We will be able to understand DS not only in terms of its aetiology, trisomy 21, but also in terms of its consequences for individuals and their intellectual and behavioural functioning.
- Specificity represents the basis for the design of specialised intervention measures that permit the creation of strategies and of more effective and direct therapeutic, learning or rehabilitation methods, to palliate or compensate for the limitations that affect persons of all ages with DS.
- Specificity is the principle that establishes scientifically the existence of associations that affect a given syndrome – in this case DS. Without specificity there would be no reason for the existence of a specialised associative movement, separate from the movement that supports people with mental retardation in general.

DEFINITION AND LEVELS OF SPECIFICITY

Specificity is 'that which is intrinsic to something that has particular characteristics', 'the particular characteristic that pertains to an entity', 'that which characterises and distinguishes one entity from another'. In the opinion of the editors of this book, work on specificity should focus on two levels:

- the level of *individual characteristics* or symptoms (Perera 1995)
- the *systemic* level – in other words, considering the relationships between characteristics or symptoms (Rondal et al. 1995)

The first level refers to the characteristics – *pathognomonic* characteristics – that correspond exclusively to a pathological category and facilitate its diagnosis. It is currently unclear whether nonaetiological pathognomonic categories exist in DS although some medical data (concerning coeliac disease for example) are very close to being pathognomonic (Bonamico et al. 2001). However, so far no evidence has been put forward to support the genetic relationship between coeliac disease and chromosome 21. Moreover, chromosomal nondisjunction and other anomalies aetiologically associated with DS are common in mental retardation of genetic origin (Shprintzen 1997). However, the two gene categories recently discovered in chromosome 21 (dosage-sensitive and nondosage sensitive genes) and the triplication of functional conserved nongenetic sequences (CNGS) that may contribute to the DS phenotype also appear to support the pathognomonic model.

The scientific analysis of mental retardation needs to take the aetiological dimension into account. For theoretical and clinical reasons it would be appropriate to explore the various types of mental retardation in greater depth, starting with those of genetic origin and, from a firmer empirical standpoint, determine which characteristics differentiate one from the other, to what extent and which signs can be found in some or in all syndromes (Rondal et al. 2003).

The perspective of specificity would appear to be clearer at the systemic level. Recent research has discovered a significant number of symptomatic characteristics in DS, which together present a specific clinical profile of the syndrome (some authors have used the term 'partial specificity' – Dykens et al. 2000). This takes us further from the notion of syndrome, typically defined as a set of symptoms characteristic of a pathological entity without the need for these characteristics to be pathognomonic or to be restricted to a given number of entities.

An interesting issue regarding DS (as with other symptoms of mental retardation, especially of genetic origin) is the task of defining, in the greatest detail possible, *syndromic specificity*. This has basic implications for mental retardation and must be carried out taking into account the global nature of personality and neurobehavioural aspects, health, susceptibility to ageing and other variables such as inclusion at school, in the family and on a social level, family or affective relationships and sexual development.

The key methodological dimension for the study of specificity must centre on intersyndromic comparison as we cannot discuss the particularities of a syndrome without making systematic comparisons with other syndromes. It is appropriate to make a list of a series of empirical indications that appear to support the specificity argument.

SPECIFICITY FROM A GENETIC PERSPECTIVE

The 33 000 (or so) genes of the human genome have been mapped in recent years and we are progressively learning more about the connections between genetic code and its consequences for health and behaviour.

In the mid-1970s geneticists studied chromosomes by means of the cytogenetic karyotype technique. Later, the ability to dye the chromosomes with gradient bands of colour allowed the different parts of each chromosome to be identified. Even more recently, techniques have been developed that allow the chemical identification of each gene (Jorde et al. 1997).

Thanks to these new techniques it is now possible to determine the presence or absence of a small area (or genetic region) in the chromosome and it will soon be possible to determine, for all individuals, if all 33 000 (or so) genes are present in their 23 pairs of chromosomes. Even now, to diagnose certain disorders such as Williams syndrome (WS), for example, one can see small microdeletions in genes by means of the fluorescence *in situ* hybridisation (FISH) technique and other molecular biological techniques (Pober & Dyckens 1996). These new molecular techniques allow the detection of microdeletions that could not have been observed with the old cytogenetic techniques.

New genetics allows us to identify cases in which genetic material is increased, decreased or changed, thus allowing us to understand the origin of the genetic change process and subsequently observe the final consequence of this process: the disorder that appears in a series of genetic conditions. We obviously still need to know what is going on meanwhile but this will require more time.

Two categories of genes exist in chromosome 21: dosage sensitive and non-dosage-sensitive genes. Only the former have an effect on the phenotype, when they are present in three copies. The effect on the phenotype can be direct or indirect. The indirect effect could be due to the interaction with genes or gene products of other chromosomes. Their effect on the phenotype may be allele specific and have a threshold effect. Finally, a triplication of certain conserved functional nongenic sequences (CNGs) might contribute the DS phenotype.

To complicate this very complex picture, the hypothesis of overexpression of the genes that are present in three copies has been partially challenged in the partial trisomy mouse model, showing that only a fraction of genes are overexpressed at the theoretical value whereas others are not overexpressed or are expressed at levels differing greatly from the expected values (Antonarakis et al. 2005).

Wisniewski, in Chapter 2 of this book, explains that recent research suggests that the DS phenotype cannot be explained by a single overexpression of genes located on trisomic chromosome 21 (the so-called gene-dosage effect). Some of the genes on chromosome 21 are not overexpressed but show normal or decreased expression in DS individuals in comparison with normal controls. At the same time, altered expression of genes located on chromosomes other than 21 have been reported in DS subjects. Thus, it appears that DS phenotype can be regarded as an outcome of altered gene and protein homeostasis resulting from abnormal gene-gene and protein-protein interactions.

Rasore Quartino, in Chapter 4, analyses the subject in depth and arrives at the following conclusion: 'The complex pattern of clinical manifestations in DS represents a peculiar feature, because, although each component can often be found in other conditions, their sum pertains only to trisomy 21.'

Moving from the gene to the final result, we gradually come closer to being able to *specify* 'what leads to what' (Hodapp & Dykens 2003). Which gene or group of genes predisposes an individual to an early onset of Alzheimer's disease, diabetes, hypertension or obesity? Which genes provoke the genetic predisposition to alcoholism or to a given personality or characteristic at the limit between the biological and the behavioural (Plomin & Rende 1991)? How do genes and genetic disorders influence the health or behaviour of persons with DS?

With regard to the so-called probabilistic model of behavioural genotypes, Dykens (1995) asserts that although many individuals with a specific intellectual disability of genetic origin present the behaviour or behaviours that are 'characteristic' of this syndrome, it is not often that they present all of these behaviours. Neither do all individuals present such behaviours to the same degree or even at the same time in their development. This is because an *intra-syndrome variability* exists within each genetically derived intellectual disability syndrome. Moreover, he affirms that certain behaviours or groups of behaviours are seen more frequently in a specific genetic syndrome than in general disability. It is not clear to what extent the characteristics or behaviours appear in one syndrome only or in more than one syndrome (Hodapp & Dykens 2004).

The connections between genetic syndromes and specific consequences at times appear to be unique whereas at other times they do not (Hodapp 1997). In the first case, that of a specific pattern, the genetic syndrome frequently provokes a particular result that is not seen in other genetic syndromes.

In fact, and up until now, the following behaviours appear to be specific to a single syndrome:

- hyperphagia (eating to excess) in Prader-Willi syndrome (Dykens 1999)
- the 'cat cry' in 5P syndrome (Gersh et al. 1995)
- the intense self-mutilation of Lesch-Nyhan syndrome (Anderson & Ernst 1994)
- picking at the body (Finucane et al. 1994) and the placing of objects in the body's orifices (Greenburg et al. 1996) in Smith-Magenis syndrome

There are probably only a few more cases in which the genetic disorder is unique in its behavioural effects. Flynt & Yule (1994) also observed this peculiarity declaring as unique only the self-stimulation behaviour in Lesch-Nyhan syndrome, the excessive eating and abnormal anxiety regarding food in Prader-Willi syndrome and the wringing of hands in Rett syndrome.

In other cases, two or more genetic disorders share characteristics or behaviours related to the aetiology. For example, children with fragile X syndrome (FXS) (Dykens et al. 1987 and Kemper 1998) and children with Prader-Willi syndrome (Dykens et al. 1992) present a unique and advantageous form of simultaneous processing (similar to Gestalt) instead of sequential processing.

THE PRACTICAL CLINICAL FOCUS OF SPECIFICITY

If we leave the genetic and aetiological aspects to one side and concentrate on the *clinical field*, focusing on DS, we will find data concerning specificity, which are explained and analysed in detail in each chapter of this book. I would like to emphasise certain findings that are especially relevant.

LANGUAGE

Rondal, in Chapter 7, explains that language in persons with DS, despite not presenting characteristics that are not found in other syndromes, displays certain characteristics that can be grouped together at the systemic specificity level. For example, it has been demonstrated that the speech and language of these individuals present acute and persistent deficiencies in form and some preserved semantic and pragmatic skills. Comparing the language of individuals with DS with skills typical of other syndromes (Rondal et al. 2004) reveals much. For example, people with WS possess a linguistic profile that is almost the opposite of that of persons with DS, displaying, for example, more skill with respect to form but strong pragmatic limitations. In FXS the typical linguistic profile is 'intermediate' between DS and WS, with phonetic-phonological difficulties (different from those found in DS), dysrythmia, perseverations, morpho-syntactic and discursive limitations, a better preserved lexical development and practical limitations.

MEMORY

Particular patterns of development and functional profiles have begun to emerge in research on memory. These patterns refer to several memory registers in DS, such as short-term memory and working memory, long-term memory, episodic and procedural or implicit memory, in contrast with other syndromes such as WS (Vicari et al. 2000; Devenny et al. 2004; Jarrold 2004).

Devenny, in Chapter 6, explains with much nuance and precision, that memory in adolescents and young adults with DS shows a characteristic profile. Implicit memory (memory for procedures and for experiences that do not require deliberate or effortful cognitive processes) and semantic memory (memory for the meanings of words and for knowledge) appear to be commensurate with their overall level of functioning. Working memory (temporary maintenance and manipulation of information) appears to be more severely impaired for auditory-verbal material than for visuo-spatial material. Episodic memory (memory for events located in a specific time and place) spans a longer duration than working memory and is impaired in both the verbal and spatial domains.

These specific strengths and weaknesses in memory are characteristic of a DS phenotype, although the biological basis for the profile is not clear at this time. In general, memory ability is related to developmental and experiential changes in the nervous system and is sensitive to the rate and characteristics of development in other domains (such as language and cognition). The memory profile associated with DS, then, will be modified across the lifespan, depending on the interaction of many developmental processes and life experiences, some of which are unique to this syndrome. In addition to systematic developmental changes, within any group of individuals with DS there is considerable variability in performance on memory and other cognitive tasks, making it difficult to predict performance capabilities and the trajectory of development of any specific individual. Understanding the sources of this variability will be critical in revealing relationships between memory processes and cognition in individuals with DS (Jarrold & Baddeley 1997; Chapman & Hesketh 2000; Vicari et al. 2000; Farran & Jarrold 2003).

Memory is responsive to life experiences, so within this system there is the possibility for modification through intervention. It is important that research first address issues related to the fundamental processes of memory in individuals with DS and their interactions with other components of cognition and then develop remediation programmes to facilitate compensation for areas of deficit.

NEUROPSYCHOLOGICAL SPECIFICITY

When analysing the psychological phenotype of DS, two things should be considered: firstly, the general deficit in intelligence and cognition and, secondly, the specific problems observed in DS that differentiate it from other forms of mental retardation.

Nadel, in Chapter 5, declares that as far as the general defect is concerned, one can consider explanations at both the neural and psychological level. Neurobiological issues include the possibility of general defects in synaptic plasticity, in impulse conduction and so on. Psychological issues include the possibility of defects in motivation, attention, aspects of learning and memory and more. He discusses current evidence concerning both of these domains.

More critical to future understanding of DS and the possibility of developing targeted treatments is an analysis of the aspects of the neuropsychological phenotype that distinguish it from other syndromes, such as WS, FXS and others (Bellugi et al. 1999; Kates et al. 2002; Bauman & Kemper 1985). These important differences in the neuropathology observed across various mental retardation syndromes strongly suggest that cognitive defects observed in these syndromes should also differ, with each syndrome demonstrating a specific pattern of spared and impaired function.

PERSONALITY

For decades, researchers and practitioners have attempted to find evidence for a personality stereotype in individuals with DS that includes a pleasant, affectionate, and passive behaviour style. However, a more nuanced exploration of personality motivation in DS reveals complexity beyond this pleasant stereotype, including reports of a less persistent motivational orientation and an overreliance on social behaviours during cognitively challenging tasks (Pitcairn & Wishart 1994; Ruskin et al. 1994; Vlachou & Farrel 2000; Kasari & Freeman 2001).

Fidler, in Chapter 9, presents the hypothesis that this personality-motivation profile observed in individuals with DS emerges as a result of the cross-domain relations between more primary (cognitive, social-emotional) aspects of the DS behavioural phenotype. Young children with DS show a general profile of delays in the development of instrumental thinking coupled with emerging relative strengths in social-emotional functioning. If it is true that a less persistent motivational orientation emerges as a secondary phenotypic result of primary strengths in social functioning and deficits in instrumental (means-end) thinking, it should be possible to alter the developmental trajectory of this personality-motivation profile with targeted and time-sensitive intervention. Important implications may arise from this regarding the planning of the intervention because, although the suggested techniques remain unproven by empirical studies at this time, continued research in this area may yield more definitive support for these suggestions. It is likely that promoting motivational development in individuals with DS with targeted and time-sensitive techniques will be effective and may affect development beyond simply improving adaptation. Helping young children with DS to recognise their own ability to generate effective strategies may lead to improved instrumental functioning and may serve to improve academic performance, independence skills, and outcomes in adulthood.

AGEING

The topic of ageing in DS is becoming increasingly important due to the notable increase in the life expectancy of persons with DS. Do those with DS generally age quicker than karyotypically normal persons? Do individuals with DS run a greater risk of contracting an Alzheimer-type pathology? Patterson examines these questions in Chapter 3 and reaches important conclusions:

Current estimates are that at least 25% of individuals with DS will develop Alzheimer-like dementia before the age of 60. It is not clear whether all those with DS will develop Alzheimer's disease if they live long enough. Moreover, all individuals with DS will develop the neuropathology associated with Alzheimer's disease: plaques and tangles. In addition, individuals with DS appear to lose functional cholinergic neurons as they age, a feature also important in Alzheimer's disease. Recent studies suggest that persons with DS are subject to lifelong elevated oxidative stress. This is significant in light of the free radical theory of ageing. These observations have led to ongoing clinical trials of antioxidants and acetylcholinesterase inhibitors to delay cognitive decline and to improve cognitive ability. Recently, studies on animal models suggest that oxidative stress is associated with cognitive decline and that regimens that ameliorate oxidative stress may also ameliorate cognitive decline with age. Of particular interest are studies of a mouse model of DS, the Ts65Dn mouse. This mouse is trisomic for many genes located on human chromosome 21. The Ts65Dn mouse shows loss in functional cholinergic neurons with age and a simultaneous loss in learning and memory. Patterson details recent attempts to ameliorate the age-dependent loss in learning and memory in these mice, and hypothesises that these mice show alterations in oxidative stress and mitochondrial function.

Other cognitive and personality dimensions are being investigated on an intersyndromic level (see various chapters of Dykens et al. 2000 and Rondal et al. 2004).

BIOMEDICAL SPECIFICITY

Biomedical research offers a number of observations that indicate significant neurological differences between genetic syndromes that may be relevant in explaining the different cognitive and linguistic functions of different phenotypes. The functional differences between DS, WSA and FXS could correspond to a syndromic variation at the cerebral level (Bellugi et al. 1990; Galaburda et al. 1994; Wisniewsky & Kida 1994; Hagerman 1996; Atkinson et al. 1997; Reiss et al. 2000). There has been much discussion on sensorial susceptibilities and limitations in persons with DS, which have been confirmed in recent studies. These include cardiac malformation and failure, hypothyroidism, auditory and visual problems, coeliac disease, leukaemia, obesity and vitamin deficiency (Rosner & Lee 1972; Weinstein 1978; Cominetti et al. 1985; Storm 1990; Pueschel & Pueschel 1992; Pueschel 1995a, 1995b; Bonamico et al. 1996; Luke et al. 1996; Franceschi et al. 1998).

It appears that there exists a particular susceptibility – perhaps close to pathognomonic, although more data are needed – in persons with DS with respect to chronological age (Van Buggenhout et al. 2000) and cognitive age (Brown 1985; Prasher 1996; Moss et al. 2000; Ribes & Sanny 2000) and in a significant portion of these persons with respect to Alzheimer-type neurodegenerative disease (Dalton & Crapper-McLachlan 1984; Kledaras et al. 1989; Lai & Williams 1989; Wisniewski & Silverman 1996, 1999; Zigman et al. 1997; Rondal et al. 2003; Wisniewski & Albertini 2004).

In Chapter 4, Rasore Quartino offers a precise examination of the biomedical pathology present in DS, a series of specific biomedical characteristics that, in comparison with the general population, in some cases increase in frequency (congenital heart defects, gastrointestinal malformations, leukaemia, autoimmune disorders, muscular hypotonia, reduced growth, early ageing) and are reduced in other cases (solid cancer, asthma) or appear with a different expression (congenital heart defects, response to therapy in leukaemia) or are present only in DS (transient leukaemia).

CONCLUSIONS

We faced the huge task of defining and documenting, by means of systematic intersyndromic comparisons, possible syndrome specificity in syndromes that include mental retardation. The end product, in the long term, may resemble a two-way mega matrix: the syndrome and neurological behaviour as coordinates and generalities of specificity as end products.

The practical implications of this investigative route are very important as therapeutic and intervention policy depend on a precise definition of what is specific and what is more generalised in the phenotype of syndromes with mental retardation. *The proposal is that the specific aspects require particular intervention methods and the nonspecific aspects require more general methods that can applied to several entities.*

It would seem that current research is inclined toward the existence of a syndromic specificity in the cognitive, behavioural, medical and even personality and social aspects of DS.

However, we have also said that knowledge of the specific characteristics of DS is the foundation upon which *the design of specific and specialised intervention measures are based*, which will permit the creation of more effective and direct strategies, therapeutic methods and learning methods to relieve or compensate for the limitations that affect persons of all ages with DS in the dimensions of cognition, language, learning, behaviour and health. For this reason Guazzo (Chapter 10), Spiker (Chapter 11) and Soresi, Nota and Ferrari (Chapter 12) have concentrated on the practical aspect of intervention in the context of early intervention, education and family and contribute suggestions of great interest.

We have also pointed out that specificity *is the criterion that scientifically supports the associative movement with respect to DS* around the world (Perera 1995). Without specificity, there is no reason to justify the existence of an associative movement different from the movement concerned with persons with nonspecific mental retardation.

Specificity leads to *specialisation*, another significant factor present in modern life that can be found in science, art, commerce and so forth – and also in the care of persons with mental retardation.

The criterion of specialisation will become more valid as knowledge and research on a given syndrome (in our case DS) increases and becomes more rigorous.

Experience tells us that the DS associations started to appear around the world because families could not obtain appropriate and specialised responses to the specific needs of their children with DS from associations for persons with nonspecific mental retardation. Moreover there is another compelling reason: the numerical significance of the group. Approximately 5 000 000 persons with DS around the world; is this number not high enough to merit their specific therapy, organisation and infrastructure without having to depend on anyone else? For this reason, specificity, the need for specialisation, is leading toward the independence of DS associations from associations that attend persons with nonspecific mental retardation.

In conclusion, and to avoid misunderstandings, I would like to stress what specificity, in practical terms, *is not*.

Specificity is not denying the many things that are common to DS and other syndromes or to nonspecific mental retardation. It is clear that there are many common elements that we know how to exploit and that we have no problem recognising.

Specificity does not mean segregating persons with DS from the rest of the population, whether they have mental retardation or not. Nor does it mean creating ghettos for persons with DS, or creating *exclusive* centres or services for persons with DS, especially for adults. When these exist, they are the exceptions that prove the rule and are normally organised as centres for research – resources for integration support (Perera 1996).

No one has said that a youth with DS cannot work, have an education or occupy an assisted dwelling with other youths, with or without mental retardation. Moreover, maintaining specific services just for persons with DS, goes against the principle of integration (Perera 2003).

What we do say, however, is that the provision of services at all levels – medical, scholastic, occupational, social – should be undertaken with specific programmes that take into account the peculiarities of DS and that specific care should also be extended to the ordinary services in our community.

There is considerable *variability* among individuals with DS (determined by the peculiar genetic load) and enormous *differences*. However, this is not an obstacle to the detection, investigation and description of a relatively homogeneous series of characteristics that are conducive to the specific study of this pathology, or to the development of more effective and direct intervention and education measures to relieve or compensate for their limitations.

Specific care for persons with DS, over the last 15 years, has helped to change the image of persons with DS and create an optimistic outlook. This specific care has already translated into:

• greater life expectancy
• better health
• better intellectual functioning
• more skill and responsibility to carry out useful, paid work

- a greater level of autonomy and independence to steer their future
- a greater capacity to live a life that is fully integrated into the community (Perera 1999)

Consequently, specificity must be the new therapeutic focus for attending to persons with DS and, in the not-too-distant future, we must ensure that the first quality criterion in the provision and evaluation of educational and social services to persons with mental retardation is that of specificity – and that other commercial criteria referring to management (taken from the business world) that have nothing to do with providing a response to the specific needs of each person with mental retardation are not applied. This book will, without doubt, help to achieve these objectives.

REFERENCES

Anderson, L., Ernst, M. (1994) Self-injury in Lesch–Nyan disease. *J Autism Develop Disord*, **24**, 67–81.
Antonarakis, S. E., Lyle, R., Dermitzakis, E. T., Reymond, A., Deutsch, S. (2005) Chromosome 21 and Down Syndrome: from genomics to pathophysiology. *Nature*, **5**, 725–738.
Atkinson, J., King, J., Braddick, O., Nokes, L., Anker, S., Braddick, K. F. (1997) A specific deficit of dorsal stream function in Williams syndrome. *Neuroreport*, **8**, 1919–1922,
Bauman, M., Kemper, T. L. (1985) Histoanatomic observations of the brain in early infantile autism. *Neurology*, **35**, 866–874.
Bellugi, U., Bihrle, A., Jemigan, T., Trauner, D., Doherty, S. (1990) Neuropsychological, neurological and neuroanatomical profile of Williams syndrome. *Am J Med Genet Suppl*, **6**, 115–125.
Bellugi, U., Lichtenberger, L., Mills, D., Galaburda, A., Korenberg, J. R. (1999) Bridging cognition, the brain and molecular genetics: evidence from Williams Syndrome. *Trends in Neuroscience*, **22**, 197–207.
Bonamico, M., Mariani, P., Rasore-Qartino, A., Scartezzini, P., Cerruti, P., Tozzi, M. C., et al. (1996) Down syndrome and celiac disease: usefulness of antigladim and antiendomysium antibodies. *Acta Paediatr*, **85**, 1503–1505.
Bonamico, M., Mariani, P., Danesi, H. M., Crisogianni, M., Failla, P., Gemme, G., Rasore Quartino, A., et al. (2001) Prevalence and clinical picture of celiac disease in Italian Down syndrome patients: a multicenter study. *J Pediatr Gastroenterol Nutr*, **33**, 139–143.
Brown, W. (1995) Genetics and aging. In M. Janicki, H. Wisniewski (eds) *Aging and Developmental Disabilities: Issues and Approaches*. Baltimore MD: Brookes, pp. 185–194.
Chapman, R. S., Hesketh, L. (2000) The behavioural phenotype of Down syndrome. *Mental Retardation and Developmental Disabilities Research Review*, **6**, 84–95.
Carr, J. (1995) *Down Syndrome: Children Growing Up*. Cambridge: Cambridge University Press.

Cominetti, M., Rasore-Quartino, A., Acutis, M. S., Vignola, G. (1985) Neonato con syndrome di Down e leucemia mieliniche acute. Difficoltá diagnostiche tra forma maligna e sindrome mieloproliferativa. *Pathologica*, **77**, 625–630.

Dalton, A., Crapper-Maclachlan, D. E. (1984) Incidence of memory deterioration in aging persons with Down syndrome. In J. Berg (ed.) *Perspectives and Progress in Mental Retardation: Biomedical Aspects*, vol. 2. Baltimore MD: University Park Press, pp. 55–62.

Devenny, D., Kittler, P., Sliwinski, M., Krinsky-McHale, S. (2004) Episodic memory across the lifespan of adults with Down syndrome. In J. A. Rondal, A. Rasore-Quartino, S. Soresi (eds) *The Adult with Down Syndrome*. London: Whurr, pp. 125–135.

Dykens, E. M. (1999) Prader-Willi Syndrome. In H. Tager-Flusberg (ed.) *Neurodevelopmental Disorders*. Cambridge MA: MIT Press.

Dykens, E. M., Hodapp, R., Finucane, B. (2000) *Genetics and Mental Retardation Syndromes*. Baltimore MD: Brookers.

Dykens, E. M., Hodapp, R., Leckman, J. F. (1987) Strengths and weakness in intellectual functioning of males with fragile X Syndrome. *Am J Ment Defic*, **92**, 234–236.

Dykens, E. M., Hodapp, R., Walsh, K. K., Nasch, L. Profiles, correlates and trajectories of intelligence in Prader-Willi syndrome. *American Academy of Child and Adolescent Psychiatry*, **31**, 1125–1130.

Farran, E. K., Jarrold, C. (2003) Visuospatial cognition in Williams Syndrome: reviewing and accounting for the strengths and weakness in performance. *Dev Neuropsychol*, **12**, 172–200.

Finucane, B. M., Konar D., Haas-Givler, B., Kurtz, M. D., Scott, L. I. (1994) The spasmodic upperbody squeeze: a characteristic behaviour in Smith-Magenis Syndrome. *Develop Med Child Neurol*, **36**, 78–83.

Flynt, J., Yule, W. (1994) Behavioural phenotypes. In M. Rutter, E. Taylor, D. L. Hersov (eds) *Child and Adolescent Psychiatry: Modern Approaches*, 3rd edn. London: Blackwell Scientific.

Franceschi, C., Chiricolo, M., Licastro, F., Zanotti, M. M., Fabris, V. (1988) Oral zinc supplementation in Down syndrome. Restoration of thymic endocrine activity and some immune defects. *J Ment Defic Res*, **32**, 169–181.

Galaburda, A., Wang, P., Bellugi, U., Rosen, M. (1994) Cytoarchitectonic anomalies in a genetically based disorder: Williams syndrome. *Cognitive Neuroscience and Neuropsychology*, **5**, 753–757.

Greenberg, F., Lewis, R. A., Potocki, L., Glaze, D., Parke, J., Killian, J. M., et al. (1996) Multidisciplinary clinical study of Smith-Magenis syndrome (deletion 17 p 11.2). *Am J Med Genet*, **62**, 247–254.

Gersh, M., Goodart, S. A., Pasztor, L. M., Harris, D. J., Weiss, L., Overhauser, J. (1995) Evidence for a distinct region causing a cat-like cry in patients with 5 p-Deletions. *Am J Hum Genet*, **56**, 1404–1410.

Hagerman, R. (1996) Biomedical advances in developmental psychology: the case of fragile X syndrome. *Dev Psychol*, **32**, 416–424.

Hodapp, R. M. (1997) Direct and indirect behavioural effects of different genetic disorders of mental retardation. *Am J Ment Retard*, **102**, 67–69.

Hodapp, R. M., Dykens, E. M. (2003) Studying behavioural phenotypes: issues, benefits, challenges. In E. Emerson, C. Hatton, T. Parmenter, T. Thompson (eds)

International Handbook of Applied Research in Intellectual Disabilities. New York: John Wiley & Sons.

Hodapp, R. M., Dykens, E. M. (2004) Genetic and behavioural phenotypes in mental retardation. In J. A. Rondal, R. M. Hodapp, S. Soresi, E. M. Dykens, L. Nota (eds) *Intellectual Disabilities: Genetics, Behaviour, Inclusion*. London: Whurr Publishers.

Jarrold, C., Baddeley, A. D. (1997) Short-term memory for verbal and visuospatial information in Down's syndrome. *Cognit Neuropsychiatry*, **2**, 101–122.

Jarrold, C. (2004) Short-term and long-term learning in Down Syndrome. In J. A. Rondal, A. Rasore Quartino, S. Soresi (eds) *The Adult with Down Syndrome*. London: Whurr Publishers.

Jorde, L. B., Carey, J. C., White, R. L. (1997) *Medical Genetics*. Saint Louis MO: Mosby.

Kasari, C., Freeman, S. F. N. (2001) Task-related social behaviour in children with Down syndrome. *Am J Ment Retard*, **106**, 253–264.

Kates, W. R., Folley, B. S., Lauham, D. C., Capone, G. T., Kaufmann, W. E. (2002) Cerebral growth in fragile X syndrome: review and comparison with Down syndrome. *Microsc Res Tech*, **57**, 159–167.

Kemper, M. B., Hagerman, R. J., Altshul-Stark, D. (1998) Cognitive profiles of boys with fragile X Syndrome. *Am J Med Genet*, **30**, 191–200.

Kledaras, J., McIlvane, W., Mackay, H. (1989) Progressive decline of picture naming in an aging Down syndrome man with dementia. *Perceptual and motor skills*, **69**, 1091–1100.

Lai, F., Williams, R. (1989) A prospective view of Alzheimer disease in Down syndrome. *Arch Neurol*, **46**, 849–853.

Luke, A., Sutton, M., Scholler, D. A., Roizen, N. J. (1996) Nutrient intake an obesity in prepubescent children with Down syndrome. *J Am Diet Assoc*, **96**, 1262–1267.

Moss, S., Tomoeda, D., Bayles, K. (2000) Comparison of the cognitive-linguistic profiles of Down syndrome adults with and without dementia to individuals with Alzheimer disease. *Journal of Medical Speech-Language Pathology*, **8**(2), 69–81.

Perera, J. (1995) *Síndrome de Down. Aspectos específicos*. Madrid: Masson.

Perera, J. (1996) Social and labour integration of people with Down syndrome. In J. A. Rondal, J. Perera, L. Nadel, A. Comblain (eds) *Down's Syndrome Psychological, Psychobiological and Socioeducational Perspectives*. London: Whurr Publishers, pp. 219–233.

Perera, J. (1999) People with Down syndrome: quality of life and future. In J. A. Rondal, J. Perera, L. Nadel (eds) *Down Syndrome. A Review of Current Knowledge*. London: Whurr Publishers, pp. 9–26.

Perera, J. (2003) *Síndrome de Down. Programa de acción educativa*, 5th edn. Madrid: Cepe.

Pitcairn, T. K., Wishart, J. G. (1994) Reactions of young children with Down's syndrome to an impossible task. *Br J Dev Psychol*, **12**, 485–489.

Plomin, R., Rende, R. (1991) Human behavioural genetics. *Annu Rev Psychol*, **42**, 161–190.

Pober, B. R., Dykens, E. M. (1996) Williams syndrome an overview of medical cognitive and behavioural features. *Child Adolesc Psychiat Clin N Am*, **5**, 929–943.

Prasher, V. (1996) Age-associated functional decline in adults with Down syndrome. *Eur J Psychiatr*, **10**, 129–135.

Pueschel, S. (1995a) Características físicas de las personas con síndrome de Down. In J. Perera (ed.) *Síndrome de Down: Aspectos específicos*. Madrid: Masson, pp. 53–63.

Pueschel, S. (1995b) Atención médica de las personas con síndrome de Down. In J. Perera (ed.) *Síndrome de Down: Aspectos específicos*. Madrid: Masson, pp. 65–73.

Pueschel, S., Pueschel, J. K. (1992) Biochemical concerns in persons with Down syndrome. Baltimore MD: Brookes.

Reiss, A., Eliez, J., Schmitt, E., Straus, E., Lai, F., Jones, W., et al. (2000) Neuroanatomy of William syndrome: a high-resolution MRI study. *J Cognit Neurosci*, **12**, 65–73.

Ribes, R., Sanny, J. (2000) Declive cognitivo en memoria y lenguaje: indicadores del proceso de envejecimiento psicológico en la persona con síndrome de Down. *Revista Síndrome de Down*, **17**, 54–59.

Rondal, J. A. (1995) Especificidad sistémica del lenguaje en el Síndrome de Down. In J. Perera (ed.) *Síndrome de Down. Aspectos específicos*. Madrid: Masson.

Rondal, J. A., Elbouz, M., Ylieff, M., Docquier, L. (2003) Françoise, a fifteen-year follow up. *Down Syndrome*, **8**(3), 89–99.

Rondal, J. A., Hodapp, R. M., Soresi, S., Dykens, E., Nota, L. (2004) *Intellectual Disabilities: Genetics, Behaviour and Inclusion*. London: Whurr Publishers.

Rosner, F., Lee, S. L. (1972) Down's syndrome and acute leukaemia: myeloblastic or lymphoblastic. Report of forty-three cases and review of the literature. *Am J Med*, **53**, 203–214.

Ruskin, E. M., Kasari, C., Mundy, P., Sigman, M. (1994) Attention to people and toys during social and object mastery in children with Down syndrome. *Am J Ment Retard*, **99**, 103–111.

Shprintzen, R. (1997) *Genetic Syndromes and Communication Disorders*. San Diego CA: Singular.

Storm, W. (1990) Hypercarotenemia in children with Down syndrome. *J Ment Defic Res*, **34**, 283–286.

Van Buggenhout, G., Lukusa, T., Trommelen, J., De Bal, C., Hamel, B., Fryns, J. P. (2000) Une étude pluridisciplinaire du syndrome de Down dans une population résidentielle d'arriérés mentaux d'âge avancé. Implications pour la suivi médical. *Journal de la trisomie*, **21**(2), 7–13.

Vicari, S., Bellucci, S., Carlesimo, G. A. (2000) Implicit and explicit memory: a functional dissociation in persons with Down syndrome. *Neuropsychologia*, **38**, 240–251.

Vlachou, M., Farrell, P. (2000) Object mastery motivation in pre-school children with and without disabilities. *Educ Psychol*, **20**, 167–176.

Weinstein, J. (1978) Congenital leukaemia and the neonatal myeloproliferative disorders associated with Down syndrome. *Clinical Haematology*, **7**, 145–147.

Wisniewski, K., Kida, E. (1994) Abnormal neurogenesis and synaptogenesis in Down syndrome brain. *Development Brain Dysfunction*, **17**, 1–12.

Wisniewski, K., Kida, E., Albertini, G. (2004) Down syndrome and Alzheimer disease. In J. A. Rondal, A. Rasore Quartino, S. Soresi (eds) *The Adult with Down Syndrome*. London: Whurr, pp. 99–111.

Wisniewski, H., Silverman, W. (1996) Alzheimer disease, neuropathology and dementia in Down syndrome. In J. A. Rondal, J. Perera, L. Nadel, A. Comblain (eds) *Down Syndrome: Psychological, Psychobiological and Socio-educational Perspectives*. London: Whurr, pp. 43–52.

Wisniewski, K., Silverman, W. (1999) Down syndrome and Alzheimer disease: variability in individual vulnerability. In J. A. Rondal, J. Perera, L. Nadel (eds) *Down Syndrome: A Review of Current Knowledge*. London: Whurr, pp. 178–194.

Zigman, W., Schup, N., Haareman, M., Silverman, W. (1997) The epidemiology of Alzheimer disease in intellectual disability research. *J Intellect Disabil Res*, **41**, 76–80.

2 Down Syndrome: from Pathology to Pathogenesis

KRYSTYNA E. WISNIEWSKI, ELIZABETH KIDA,
ADAM A. GOLABEK, MARIUSZ WALUS, AUSMA RABE
Institute for Basic Research in Developmental Disabilities, New York, USA

SONIA PALMINIELLO, GIORGIO ALBERTINI
Ospedale San Raffaele Pisana, Rome, Italy

SUMMARY

Down syndrome (DS) is the most common birth defect associated with mental retardation. However, it remains unclear how an extra copy of chromosome 21 leads to characteristic brain abnormalities (decreased number of neurons, abnormal cortical lamination, delayed myelination, synaptic changes and early Alzheimer pathology) causing cognitive and motor dysfunction. It appears that the DS phenotype can be regarded as an outcome of altered gene and protein homeostasis resulting from abnormal gene-gene and protein-protein interactions. Our studies – and those of others – exploring protein expression patterns using a proteomic approach either in human DS tissues or in mouse models for DS provide support for this idea. The function of proteins misexpressed in the DS brain is associated with a range of biological processes such as signal transduction, morphogenesis, cellular structural organisation, apoptosis, synaptogenesis, DNA repair and diverse metabolic processes, which emphasise the unusual complexity of DS pathogenesis.

INTRODUCTION

The genetic cause of DS was unravelled by Lejeune and colleagues, who identified an extra chromosome 21 in nine affected children (Lejeune et al. 1959). Down syndrome results, in 90% to 95% of cases, from complete trisomy of chromosome 21 due to nondisjunction during gamete formation and in about 95% of cases is of maternal origin (Antonarakis 1991). Only about 2% to 4% of cases result from translocation, and 2% to 4% are caused by mosaicism (Hook 1981).

Down Syndrome: Neurobehavioural Specificity. Edited by JA Rondal and J Perera.
© 2006 John Wiley & Sons Ltd.

Down syndrome is the most common autosomal aneuploidy in humans, with incidence of around 1 in 700 to 1 in 1000 live births. The phenotypic features of DS vary. John Langdon Down noticed that, apart from mental inability, affected individuals also have circulatory problems, susceptibility to infection and low life expectancy (Down 1866). Two consistent features of DS, mental retardation and neonatal hypotonia, are associated with a wide range of other abnormalities such as congenital heart defects, gastrointestinal malformations, endocrine and hematopoietic dysfunction with transitory leukemogenic syndrome or leukaemia, growth disturbances with craniofacial abnormalities, microcephaly, short stature and seizures and psychiatric symptoms that occur with varying prevalence and intensity (Korenberg et al. 1994).

Although the cognitive level of infants with DS may be relatively high (70 to 80 standard IQ score range) standardised IQ scores show a gradual decline and are within the low-to-moderate range (average 30 to 40) by 11 years of age (Carr 1995), which reflects a low rate of development rather than a loss of skills already gained (Hauser-Cram et al. 2001). Deficits in expressive language and reduction in intelligence scores from early to middle childhood predominate, whereas nonverbal, social and play skills remain relatively strong (Sigman et al. 1999). Despite early diagnosis and early intervention, individuals with DS still function in the moderate to severe range of mental retardation during the first decades of life (Connolly et al. 1993). Furthermore, even early intervention programmes did not change the developmental delay of DS children, who typically gained about half a month of mental age for each month of chronological age (Hauser-Cram et al. 2001). However, due to better medical care, the median age at death of people with DS has increased from 25 years in 1983 to 49 years in 1997, an average increase of 1.7 years per year studied (Yang et al. 2002).

Our knowledge of the neurobiology of DS and our understanding of the morphological, biochemical and molecular bases of brain dysfunction in DS individuals is still very limited. Completion of the human genome project (Venter et al. 2001), introduction of mouse models for DS, and implementation of proteomic techniques in recent years have provided a new impact to this understanding. In general, DS research can be divided into three stages: pregenomic, genomic, and proteomic. Below, we summarise briefly and rather selectively, given the space limitations, the research findings that we believe most contribute to a better understanding of the abnormal development and function of DS brain.

PATHOLOGICAL ASPECTS

The first neuropathological descriptions of DS brain were provided many years ago (Fraser & Mitchell 1876; Davidoff 1928) but a systematic analysis of structural alterations in developing DS brain has not yet been undertaken. Most previous studies either included a small number of cases or referred to a particular brain region, selected type of pathology, or a short period of brain development. The pattern of gross pathology analysed by both neuropathological examination or, in recent years, by neuroimaging techniques is relatively well documented. The weight, configuration, gyration pattern and onset of myelination in the DS brain at 15 to 22 weeks' gestation and in newborns are similar to those of normal brain (Schmidt-Sidor et al. 1990). After 3 to 5 months of age, the differences become apparent in that DS brain often has lower weight, shortening of the anterior-posterior dimension, flattening of the occipital lobes and wide primary cortical gyri with shallow sulci and narrow superior temporal gyri (Davidoff 1928; Schmidt-Sidor et al. 1990; Wisniewski 1990). However, it should be emphasised that not all individuals with DS manifest these structural changes and not to the same degree. Interestingly, the cerebellum and the brainstem are markedly reduced in size (Crome et al. 1966; Schmidt-Sidor et al. 1990). In agreement with this, the first high-resolution magnetic resonance (MRI) study of children and young adults with DS, published recently, showed that mean total brain volume is indeed smaller in individuals with DS than in controls (by around 18%) with a disproportionately small cerebellar volume. The same MRI study also documented larger adjusted volumes of subcortical (basal ganglia), parietal, and temporal grey matter, with significantly smaller superior temporal white matter volume (Pinter et al. 2001). Significantly larger lateral ventricles and smaller whole-brain volume with smaller planum temporale was also found in a volumetric MRI study of adults with DS (Frangou et al. 1997); however, the Alzheimer-type pathology present in adults with DS (Wisniewski et al. 1985) may significantly contribute to the brain atrophy observed.

The prominent and early involvement of the cerebellum in DS brain pathology, which was also reported in mouse models for DS (Baxter et al. 2000) is of special interest given that the cerebellum controls not only muscle tone and motor coordination but, according to recent studies, also cognition, verbal fluency, and language (Ackermann et al., 1998; Schmahmann & Sherman 1998), all of which are compromised in individuals with DS. The smaller volume of the frontal lobes in some children with DS demonstrated by MRI analyses (Jernigan et al. 1993) did not reach significance in another study (Pinter et al. 2001).

Reduction of the neuronal population in various areas of the cerebral cortex in DS brain was documented by many studies (Davidoff 1928; Colon 1972; Wisniewski et al. 1984, 1986; Ross et al. 1984; Becker et al. 1986) and it involves mostly neurons of layers II and IV and, to a lesser degree, also of layer III (Ross et al. 1984; Wisniewski et al. 1984, 1986). Layers II and IV contain stellate cells exerting inhibitory actions; thus reduction of this particular neuronal population may lead to an imbalance of cortical circuits.

Differences in the development of cortical lamination between DS and controls were also reported (Golden & Hyman 1994; Wisniewski & Kida 1994); however, microdysgenesia is rather rare in DS foetuses as it was found only in four DS foetuses of 32 studied (Unterberger et al. 2003). A lower total number and density of neurons in the cochlear nuclei was also found (Gandolfi et al. 1981).

Synapses appear in the human cortex early in development and are present in foetuses at 8 weeks' gestation (Molliver et al. 1973). Synaptic plasticity is associated with learning and memory processes (Mollgaard et al. 1971). Synaptic density was similar to that in controls in the sensorimotor cortex in four autopsy DS foetuses at ages 19, 20, 23 and 36 weeks' postconception. However, at the later stages of gestation, a higher percentage of primitive and a lower percentage of intermediate contacts and reduced synaptic parameters such as presynaptic and postsynaptic length, presynaptic and postsynaptic width and cleft width was detected in DS (Petit et al. 1984). Synaptic density in layer III may be reduced at birth (Takashima et al. 1994). In agreement with this, synaptic profiles we studied in the visual cortex from birth to 18 years showed lower synaptic density at birth and in young adults with DS. Reduced presynaptic length and average surface area per synaptic contact zone were found in all age groups of individuals with DS in comparison with controls (Wisniewski et al. 1986). However, our immunocytochemical studies suggested that the pattern of synaptogenesis may be altered early in the foetal DS brain (Wisniewski & Kida 1994). In agreement with this, a recent proteomic study of DS foetuses at 19 weeks' gestation showed a significant reduction of synaptosomal markers (SNAP 25 and alpha SNAP) and dendritic spine marker (drebrin) in comparison with control foetuses (Weitzdoerfer et al. 2001). It should be mentioned here that a reduction of drebrin was not confirmed by further immunocytochemical analysis (Unterberger et al. 2003).

In the visual cortexes of eight children with DS 4 months to 5 years of age, Becker and colleagues found that the total mean dendritic length, number of intersections, number of branches, order of branching and points of maximum branching to the centre of the neuron decreased with increasing age, unlike in normal controls. Moreover, an unexpected, expanded dendritic tree in infants with DS at 4 months of age was detected. The authors suggested that this excessive early outgrowth of dendritic branches in young infants with DS may reflect a compensatory response to neuronal loss at the beginning, followed by 'premature ageing' of cells and subsequent dendritic atrophy (Becker et al. 1986). This old concept of 'premature ageing' of DS brain (Wisniewski et al. 1978, 1982) recently received fresh input from the analysis of radial cell columns in the part of Wernicke's area (Buxhoeveden et al. 2002) and Brodman areas 21 and 22 in the temporal lobe, area 40 in the parietal cortex, and area 17 in the occipital lobe of nine individuals with DS 3 to 56 years of age (Buxhoeveden and Casanova 2004). These studies showed that the size of the cell columns in individuals with DS reached adult spacing by 4 and 6 years of age in all areas examined, in contrast to age-matched controls, in which the column size was distinctly smaller in children than in adults, except for the primary visual cortex. The authors suggested that the development of the cell columns is very rapid in the association cortex but not the primary visual cortex in DS brain, thus reflecting a form of accelerated maturation.

The major sites of excitatory synaptic input to the neurons in brain tissue, which enable proper synaptic signalling, integration, and plasticity, are dendritic spines. Long-term potentiation (LTP), a candidate learning and memory mechanism, is mediated in part by changes in spine number and structure in the hippocampus. Mice lacking NMDA receptor subunits in hippocampus fail to express LTP and show impairment during learning and memory tasks, which can be overcome by enriched environment–induced increases in production of dendritic spines (Rampon et al. 2000). Dendritic spine abnormalities were reported in the hippocampus in children with DS at 8 and 9 months of age (Purpura 1975) and in four adults with DS (Ferrer & Gullota 1990). In the motor cortex of an 18-month-old child with DS, some pyramidal neurons were severely deprived of spines, whereas the others were covered by innumerable, extremely small spines with small pedicles (Marin-Padilla 1972, 1976). Dendritic spine abnormalities were also found in the visual cortex in children with DS older than 4 months of age, but not younger (Takashima et al. 1981). Small spines in neonates and elongated spines in older infants also were reported (Takashima et al. 1994). However, the dendritic tree of pyramidal neurons of layer III of the prefrontal cortex, which represents the key commissural and associative neuronal elements, showed no abnormalities in two individuals with DS (36 weeks' gestation and 2.5 postnatal month) during the perinatal period of most intensive dendritic differentiation in this area (Vukšić et al. 2002). This finding, together with the observations of Takashima et al. (1981), suggests that dendritic spine pathology appears relatively late during brain development in DS. Spine pathology occurs in various pathological conditions and many forms of mental retardation so it was proposed that it is most likely to reflect widespread neuronal loss and partial deafferentiation of the spiny neurons (for a review see Fiala et al. 2002). In this respect, the dendritic spine pathology present in DS brain, one of the potential structural bases of the cognitive dysfunction of individuals with DS, could be caused by loss of proper afferent connections as a result of neuronal loss, which has been documented in DS brain in the postnatal period.

Delay in myelination is sometimes observed in DS (Wisniewski & Schmidt-Sidor 1989). Calcification of the basal ganglia has also been documented (Wisniewski et al. 1982). Neuropathologic features of AD are a consistent finding in DS brain. The first extracellular deposits of amyloid-β peptide in the form of diffuse plaques were found in our material in a 12-year-old child with DS (Kida et al. 1995). All older persons (>30 to 40 years) with DS develop senile plaques, neurofibrillary tangles, and granulovacuolar degeneration (Jervis 1948; Wisniewski et al. 1985).

Brain cholinergic markers are normal in individuals with DS at birth (Kish et al. 1989). However, the cholinergic, noradrenergic and serotoninergic systems are compromised in the brains of adults with DS (Yates et al. 1983; Casanova et al. 1985). These changes appear to be caused by degeneration and cell loss of the cortical projection neurons arising from the nucleus basalis of Meynerti (cholinergic), locus ceruleus (noradrenergic), and dorsal raphae nuclei (serotoninergic). The loss of cholinergic function and the decrease in trkA (high-affinity NGF receptors) immunoreactivity in the basal forebrain of Ts65Dn mice, a model of DS, correlated with deficits in behavioural flexibity on a spatial task that appeared at around 6 months of age (Granholm et al. 2000).

GENETIC STUDIES

A high-quality, nearly complete sequence of chromosome 21 was published in 2000 (Hattori et al. 2000). Chromosome 21 (HSA21) is the smallest human autosome, extending for 33.8 Mb, predicted to contain 261 to 364 protein-coding genes. Analysis of the proteins encoded by genes located on HSA21 identified to date indicates that they are involved in 87 different biological processes, have 81 different molecular functions and are localised in 26 different cellular compartments. Their most common function involves DNA-binding and transcription factor activity (15 proteins); their most common localisation is the nucleus and the plasma membrane (19 and 15 proteins, respectively) and the most common biological process in which they are implicated is signal transduction (11 proteins) (Antonarakis et al. 2004). However, it should be stressed that complete genetic reannotation of HSA21 has yet to be finished and is currently in progress.

Two hypotheses have been created to explain the DS phenotype: gene dosage effect and amplified developmental instability. The first proposes that DS phenotype, like other aneuploidies, is caused by the cumulative effect of imbalance of the genes located on the triplicated chromosome (Bond & Chandley 1983). The second hypothesis predicts that DS phenotype is caused by a disturbance of chromosome balance and a disruption of homeostasis (Shapiro 1983).

After the 'gene dosage effect' hypothesis, phenotypic maps assigning particular phenotypic features to a specific region of 21q have been created by correlating the cytogenetic information from patients with a rare partial duplication of 21q with clinical phenotypes (Korenberg et al. 1994). Conceptual bases for phenotypic mapping of aneuploid syndromes have been put forth by Epstein (1993). In trisomy 21, the phenotype could be a direct consequence of a gene dosage imbalance of the genes on 21q, which are present in three copies, thus theoretically leading to an mRNA level that is 1.5 times higher than normal. As a consequence, a transcript map of a putative minimal or 'DS critical region' on 21q encompassing a 1.2 Mb region around D21S55 (Peterson et al. 1994) or a 2.5 Mb carbonyl reductase, transcription factor ERG (CBR-ERG) (Pritchard & Kola 1999) has been established.

Numerous proteins encoded by genes located on HSA21 can affect the structure or function of the brain. These proteins include amyloid-β precursor protein (APP), superoxide dismutase (SOD-1), S100β (β subunit), glutamate receptor subunit 5, cystatin B, glycinamide ribonucleotide synthetase–aminoimidazole ribonucleotide synthetase – glycinamide ribonucleotide formyltransferase protein complex, Purkinje cell protein 4, Ets-2, the DS cell-adhesion molecule (DSCAM), Down syndrome – critical region protein-1 (DSCR-1), dual-specificity tyrosine-(Y)-phosphorylation kinase (DYRK1A), synaptojanin, HMG14, intersectin (ITSN), or single-minded homolog 2 (SIM2). These proteins are involved in such important biological processes as cell-cycle kinetics, neurite outgrowth, synaptic plasticity and neuronal differentiation (DYRK1A), axonal outgrowth (DSCAM), neurotrophic activity with effect on glia and neurons (S100β), plasticity and neurite outgrowth (APP), synaptic transmission, synaptic vesicles endocytosis and signalling (synaptojanin), transcription (Ets-2), synchronised cell divisions (SIM2) or LTP/LTD (DSCR-1). Some of these proteins such as APP, DSCR-1, ITSN, S100β, SOD-1 were already found to be overexpressed in DS but some of them only at the mRNA and not at the protein level (APP, SOD-1) (for reviews see Capone 2001; Engidawork & Lubec 2003; Benavides-Piccione et al. 2004). Furthermore, at least 16 genes or predicted genes on HSA21 may be involved in mitochondrial energy generation and reactive oxygen species metabolism, and six may control gene expression by affecting folate or methyl group metabolism (for a review see Roizen & Patterson 2003).

However, it appears that the complex phenotypic presentation of DS cannot be explained on the basis of gene dosage effect alone. It was found that, in foetuses or adults with DS, a number of genes across the genome are expressed at either higher or lower transcriptional levels than normal (for a review see Jenkins & Velinov 2001). Among 78 genes present in three copies on mouse chromosome 16 analysed by RT-PCR in one of the mouse models for DS, ~37% of genes were expressed at the expected value of 1.5-fold; ~45% of the genes showed expression levels lower than 1.5; 9% were not significantly overexpressed whereas 18% had expression levels higher than 1.5 (Lyle et al. 2004). Comparison of the expression of 136 mouse orthologs of HSA21 genes in various tissues of trisomic mouse (Ts65Dn) by microarray analysis showed that the majority, but not all, of the 77 genes at dosage imbalance in trisomic mice displayed 1.5-fold increases in transcript levels and that some disomic genes were also dysregulated (Kahlem et al., 2004). However, in another microarray analysis of foetal DS brain and of astrocyte cell lines from foetal brain of DS and controls, global upregulation of chromosome 21 gene expression was disclosed (Mao et al. 2003). A few individual genes were consistently and selectively upregulated. Some of the most consistently upregulated genes included DSCR-2, SOD-1, HSP 70, ζ-crystallin, cystatin B, and ATP synthase.

A different set of genes was identified by using indexing-based differential display PCR, carried out on cultured neurospheres generated from cortices of foetal DS brain (8–18 weeks after conception) (Bahn et al. 2002). SCG10, a neuron-specific, growth-associated protein that is regulated by the non-restrictive silencer factor REST (also known as repressor element-1 silencing transcription factor), revealed a dramatic reduction of the expression level. Repression of other genes regulated by REST, such as the gene encoding the L1 cell-adhesion molecule, synapsin, and β4-tubulin as well as REST/REST1 itself, was also detected. Although APP expression was reduced, two other HSA21 genes tested – DSCR-1 and DSCAM – were upregulated. Moreover, a striking reduction of neurogenesis of cultured DS but not control stem cells and progenitor cells was observed, with a dramatically reduced number of differentiating neurons, reduction of average neurite length and with misshapen neurites with excessive side-branches and convoluted neurites. This important study, demonstrating that DS stem cells and progenitor cells show downregulation of REST, which through its target genes is involved in brain development, neuronal plasticity and synapse formation, suggests that a specific regulatory pathway of neuronal gene expression is disrupted and at an early stage of DS brain development.

The data above appear to confirm the assumption that in the DS brain the resultant pattern and timing of gene expression in cells of neuronal and glial lineage may not be determined by gene dosage effect alone and could result in complex gene-gene interactions, with consequences for brain development and function that are difficult to predict at present (Capone 2001). It was pointed out recently that there is no evidence that individual loci on HSA21 are singularly responsible for specific phenotypic abnormalities in DS and each of the phenotypic features of DS is a multifactorial trait (Shapiro 1999). A class of candidate genes that may contribute significantly to DS phenotype may also include those genes that are located on chromosomes other than HSA21 and that show altered pattern of temporal and spatial expression in DS tissues.

PROTEOMIC STUDIES

Numerous proteins involved in signalling processes such as 14-3-3 protein γ isoform, nucleoside diphosphate kinase (NDK)-B, Rab GDP-dissociation inhibitor (GDI)-β, and signalling adapter proteins as well as several transcription and translation factors, some cytoskeletal proteins such as β-tubulin or some actin-binding proteins including moesin, have decreased levels in the foetal DS brain (for a review see Engidawork & Lubec 2003). These findings confirm the notion that, in the DS brain, the expression of many genes involved in neurogenesis and proper development of the central nervous system may be disrupted.

To address this issue, as a first step to better characterise which biological processes are affected by trisomy 21 in humans, several research teams initiated the creation of two-dimensional protein maps of the DS brain by using two-dimensional electrophoresis followed by mass spectrometry identification of protein spots differentially expressed in DS *versus* control brains (Kim et al. 2000; Oppermann et al. 2000; Cheon et al. 2001; Freidl et al. 2001; Yoo et al. 2001; Gulesserian et al. 2001; Engidawork & Lubec 2001, 2003; Engidawork et al. 2003; Shin et al. 2004 – and a review, Vercauteren et al. 2004). Some of the proteins identified showed increased levels in DS foetal brain, such as double-strand break repair protein rad 21 homologue, eukaryotic translation initiation factor 3 subunit 5, mixed-lineage leukaemia septin-like fusion protein-B, heat shock protein 75 (Engidawork et al. 2003), α-tubulin (Oppermann et al. 2000), or GRP 78 (Yoo et al. 2001). The levels of other proteins were reduced, such as β-amyloid precursor-like protein 1, tropomyosin 4-anaplastic lymphoma kinase fusion oncoprotein type 2, Nck adaptor protein 2, Src homology domain growth factor receptor bound 2-like endophilin B2, β tubulin, septin 7 and hematopoietic stem/progenitor cells 140 (Engidawork et al. 2003), stathmin (Cheon et al. 2001) or thioredoxin peroxidase-I (Gulessarian et al. 2001). However, the spatial and temporal expression of these and many other gene products implicated in DS pathology in both normal and DS brain is either fragmentary or completely unknown and studies aimed at addressing these issues have only recently been initiated.

To identify proteins showing either increased or decreased levels or proteins incorrectly modified post-translationally in DS brain we perform a detailed spatial and temporal analysis of proteins differentially expressed in DS brain in comparison with controls. These proteins are separated using two-dimensional electrophoresis of brain homogenates from Ts65Dn mice followed by mass spectrometry (MS/MS) identification of differentially expressed protein spots. The level and tissue distribution of proteins differentially expressed in trisomic and control mice is afterwards verified in DS and control human brains at various pre-, peri-, and postnatal stages by using Western blotting and immunocytochemistry.

Ts65Dn mice represent one of the currently available mouse models for DS. These mice have segmental trisomy for the ~16Mb region of mouse chromosome 16 that extends from the *Mrpl* 39 to the *Znf* 295 gene and encompasses a predicted 132 genes that are homologous to those located in

21q11–21q22.13 of HSA21 (Davisson et al. 1990, Reeves et al. 1995). Ts65Dn mice demonstrate several phenotypic features of DS such as craniofacial abnormalities, reduced neuronal density in the cerebellar cortex and dentate gyrus, age-related degeneration of basal forebrain cholinergic neurons, reduction in excitatory synapses in the temporal cortex, astrogliosis, and learning and behavioural deficits (Reeves et al. 1995; Escorihuela et al. 1998; Baxter et al. 2000; Granholm et al. 2000).

There are several reasons for our decision to initiate the proteomic studies using mouse, not human, tissues. First, by using trisomic and wild-type control animals from the same litter, we substantially reduce the well-known inter-individual differences in protein expression levels. Second, due to this approach, we can eliminate post mortem artifacts associated with autolysis often encountered in autopsy human tissues. Third, this tactic allows us to eliminate several factors that may affect significantly the protein pattern such as seizures, brain oedema, brain anoxia, the effect of medication or metabolic defects, common in individuals with DS. The fact that segmental trisomy in Ts65Dn mouse does not replicate faithfully the gene content of HSA21q is our major concern. For this reason the results obtained in mouse brains must be verified using human material.

To date we have identified 21 proteins differentially expressed in trisomic mice in comparison with wild-type mice (Table 2.1). The location of some of these proteins on silver-stained gels is presented in Figure 2.1. The proteins we identified play various biological roles and are involved in numerous physiological processes. Dysregulation of some of them, such as crystallin isozyme (Mao et al. 2003), 14-3-3 (Peyrl et al. 2002), multidrug resistance protein (Engidawork et al. 2001), or glutathione S-transferase isozymes (Gulesserian et al. 2001) has already been documented in human DS brain, which validates the approach we decided to employ. Interestingly, some of the proteins we have been able to identify to date have been implicated in clinical syndromes associated with mental retardation. These proteins include carbonic anhydrase II (Shah et al. 2004) and Williams-Beuren protein homologue (Makeyev et al. 2004). Further analysis of the spatial and temporal distribution and expression of these proteins in DS brain will provide more insight into their putative role in DS pathogenesis. We believe that identification and assessment of protein expression using a proteomic approach is an important first step in understanding the molecular mechanisms leading to altered development and progressive neurodegeneration of DS brain.

ACKNOWLEDGEMENTS

The authors thank Mrs Maureen Stoddard-Marlow for copy-editing the manuscript. This work was supported by NYS Office for Mental Retardation in Developmental Disabilities and Tosinvest, Rome, Italy.

Table 2.1. Proteins differentially expressed in the brain of Ts65Dn mice in comparison with controls

Name	Gi accession no.	Chromosome location	Type of dysregulation	Major function(s)
14-3-3 (γ and δ)	14198143	5	↑[a]	control of cell cycle, growth, differentiation, survival, apoptosis, migration and spreading
Carbonic anhydrase II	115457	3	↑	respiratory gas exchange, pH homoeostasis, ion transport
Protein disulfide isomerase		11	↑	rearrangement of disulfide bonds in proteins, molecular chaperone
Tumour metastatic process associating protein	387496	11	→	metastasis-suppressor protein, nucleoside diphosphate kinase A
Carbonyl reductase 3	27413160	16	↑	carbonyl reductase (NADPH) and oxidoreductase
Multidrug resistance protein (RhoA)	307375	9	↑	signal transduction, proto-oncogene
Cytochrome c oxidase, subunit Va	6680986	9	↑	electron transport
Cytochrome c oxidase, subunit Vb	6753500	1	↑	electron transport
Dual specificity phosphatase 3	21312314	11	↑	protein tyrosine/serine/ threonine phosphatase activity, cell cycle
Ubiquitin conjugating enzyme	12838544	10	↑	putative ubiquitin-conjugating enzyme E2N
Cryab protein (α B-crystallin)	14789702	9	↑	molecular chaperone
Dynein, cytoplasmic light chain 2A	21735425	2	↑	microtubule-based movement
NADH dehydrogenase	54611544	19	↑	oxidative phosphorylation
Neurocalcin	15029877	8	↑	calcium sensor
Similar to protein kinase C inhibitor	34868506	11	→	adenosine 5-monophosphoramidase
Glutamate-ammonia ligase	31982332	1	↑	glutamine biosynthesis
Glutathione S-transferase mu1	6754084	3	↑	detoxification of electrophiles
3-phosphoglycerate dehydrogenase	56104627	3	↑	phosphoglycerate dehydrogenase
ATPaseH+ transporting V1 subunit	16758754	6	→	ATPase activity coupled to transmembrane movement of ions
Fumaryloacatoacetate hydrolase domain containing 2A	29366814	2	↑	isomerase
Williams-Beuren syndrome chromosome region 1 homologue	15808988	5	→	translation initiation factor

[a] Up or down arrows indicate either increased or decreased level of a given protein in trisomic animals in comparison with controls.

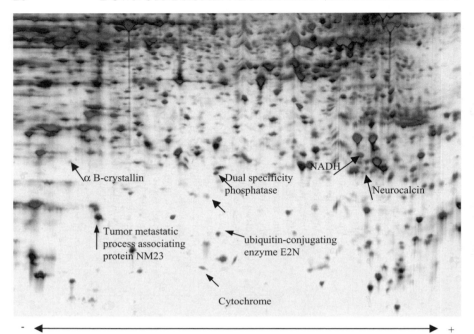

Figure 2.1. Two-dimensional gel pattern of brain proteins of 3 month-old Ts65Dn mouse. 100 µg protein was loaded onto Immobiline Dry-Strip 3–10 non-linear gradient, 18 cm, then resolved on 10% SDS-PAGE and silver-stained according to the manufacturer's protocol (Amersham). Some differentially expressed proteins are marked by arrows and labelled on presented fragment of the gel.

REFERENCES

Ackermann, H., Wildgruber, D., Daum, I., Grodd, W. (1998) Does the cerebellum contribute to the cognitive aspects of speech production? A functional magnetic resonance imaging (fMRI) study in humans. *Neurosci Lett*, **247**, 187–190.

Antonarakis, S. E. (1991) Parental origin of the extra chromosome in trisomy 21 as indicated by analysis of DNA polymorphisms. Down Syndrome Collaborative Group. *N Engl J Med*, **324**, 872–876.

Antonarakis, S. E., Lyle, R., Dermitzakis, E. T., Reymond, A., Deutsch, S. (2004) Chromosome 21 and Down syndrome: from genomics to pathophysiology. *Nat Rev Genet*, **5**, 725–738.

Bahn, S., Mimmack, M., Ryan, M., Caldwell, M. A., Jauniaux, E., Starkey, M., et al. (2002) Neuronal target genes of the neuron-restrictive silencer factor in neurospheres derived from foetuses with Down's syndrome: a gene expression study. *Lancet*, **359**, 310–315.

Baxter, L. L., Moran, T. H., Richtsmeier, J. T., Troncoso, J., Reeves, R. H. (2000) Discovery and genetic localization of Down syndrome cerebellar phenotype using the Ts65Dn mouse. *Hum Mol Genet*, **9**, 195–202.

Becker, L. E., Armstrong, D. L., Chan, F. (1986) Dendritic atrophy in children with Down's syndrome. *Ann Neurol*, **20**, 520–526.

Benavides-Piccione, R., Ballesteros-Yanez, I., de Lagran. M. M., Elston, G., Estivill, X., Fillat, C., et al. (2004) On dendrites in Down syndrome and DS murine models: a spiny way to learn. *Prog Neurobiol*, **74**, 111–126.

Bond, A. G., Chandley, A. C. (1983) *Aneuploidy*. Oxford: Oxford University Press.

Buxhoeveden, D., Casanova, M. (2004) Accelerated maturation in brains of patients with Down's syndrome. *J Intel Dis Res*, **48**, 704–705.

Buxhoeveden, D., Fobbs, A., Roy, E., Casanova, M. (2002) Quantitative comparison of radial cell columns in children with Down's syndrome and controls. *J Intel Dis Res*, **46**, 76–81.

Capone, G. T. (2001) Down syndrome: advances in molecular biology and the neurosciences. *Dev Beh Ped*, **22**, 40–59.

Carr, J. (1994) Long-term-outcome for people with Down's syndrome. *J Child Psychol Psychiatry*, **35**, 425–439.

Casanova, M. F., Walker, L. C., Whitehouse, P. J., Price, D. L. (1985) Abnormalities of the nucleus basalis in Down's syndrome. *Ann Neurol*, **18**, 310–313.

Cheon, M. S., Fountoulakis, M., Dierssen, M., Ferreres, J. C., Lubec, G. (2001) Expression profiles of proteins in foetal brain with Down syndrome. *J Neural Transm Suppl*, **61**, 311–319.

Colon, E. J. (1972) The structure of the cerebral cortex in Down syndrome. *Neuropediatrics*, **3**, 362–376.

Connolly, B. H., Morgan, S. B., Russell, F. F., Fulliton, W. L. (1993) A longitudinal study of children with Down syndrome who experienced early intervention programming. *Phys Ther*, **73**, 170–179.

Crome, L., Cowie, V., Slater, E. A. (1966) Statistical note on cerebellar and brain-stem weight in mongolism. *J Ment Defic Res*, **10**, 69–72.

Davidoff, L. (1928) The brain in Mongolian idiocy. *Arch Neurol Psychiatry*, **20**, 1229–1257.

Davisson, M. T., Schmidt, C., Akeson, E. C. (1990) Segmental trisomy for murine chromosome 16: a new system for studying Down syndrome. In D. Patterson, C. J. Epstein (eds) *Molecular Genetics of Chromosome 21 and Down Syndrome*. New York: Wiley-Liss, pp. 263–280.

Down, J. L. H. (1866) Observation on an ethnic classification of idiots. *London Hosp Clin Lect Rep*, **3**, 259–262.

Ellis, W. G., McCulloch, J. R., Corely, C. L. (1974) Presenile dementia in Down's syndrome. *Neurology*, **24**, 101–106.

Engidawork, E., Gulesserian, M., Fountoutakis, M., Lubec, G. (2003) Aberrant protein expressions in cerebral cortex of fetus with Down syndrome. *Neuroscience*, **122**, 145–154.

Engidawork, E., Lubec, G. (2001) Protein expression in Down syndrome brain. *Amino Acids*, **21**, 331–361.

Engidawork, E., Lubec, G. (2003) Molecular changes in foetal Down syndrome brain. *J Neurochem*, **84**, 895–904.

Engidawork, E., Roberts, J. C., Hardmeier, R., Scheper, R. J., Lubec, G. (2001) Expression of the multidrug resistance P glycoprotein (Pgp) and multidrug resistance associated protein (MRP1) in Down syndrome brains. *J Neural Transm Suppl*, **61**, 35–45.

Epstein, C. J. (1993) The conceptual bases for the phenotypic mapping of conditions resulting from aneuploidy. In C. Epstein (ed.) *The Phenotypic Mapping of Down Syndrome and Other Aneuploid Conditions*. New York NY: Wiley-Liss, pp. 1–18.

Escorihuela, R. M., Vallina, I. F., Martinez-Cue, C., Baamonde, C., Dierssen, M., Tobena, A., et al. (1998) Impaired short- and long-term memory in Ts65Dn mice, a model for Down syndrome. *Neurosci Lett*, **247**, 171–174.

Ferrer, I., Gullotta, F. (1990) Down's syndrome and Alzheimer's disease: dendritic spine counts in the hippocampus. *Acta Neuropathol*, **79**, 680–685.

Fiala, J. C., Spacek, J., Harris, K. M. (2002) Dendritic spine pathology cause or consequence of neurological disorders. *Brain Res Rev*, **39**, 29–54.

Fountoulakis, M. (2001) Proteomics: current technologies and application in neurological disorders and toxicology. *Amino Acids*, **21**, 363–381.

Frangou, S., Aylward, E., Warren, A., Sharma, T., Barta, P., Pearlson, G. (1997) Small planum temporale volume in Down's syndrome: a volumetric MRI study. *Am J Psychiatry*, **154**, 1424–1429.

Fraser, M., Mitchell, A. (1876) Kalmuc idiocy: report of a case with autopsy with notes on sixty-two cases. *J Ment Sci*, **22**, 169–179.

Freidl, M., Gulesserian, T., Lubec, G., Fountoulakis, M., Lubec, B. (2001) Deterioration of the transcriptional, splicing and elongation machinery in brain of foetal Down syndrome. *J Neural Transm*, **61** Suppl., 47–57.

Gandolfi, A., Horoupian, D. S., de Teresa, R. M. (1981) Pathology of the auditory system in autosomal trisomies with morphometric and quantitative study of the ventral cochlear nucleus. *J Neurol Sci*, **51**, 43–50.

Golden, J. A., Hyman, B. T. (1994) Development of the superior temporal neocortex is anomalous in trisomy 21. *J Neuropathol Exp Neurology*, **53**, 513–520.

Granholm, A.-C. E., Sanders, L. A., Crnic, L. S. (2000) Loss of cholinergic phenotype in basal forebrain coincides with cognitive decline in a mouse model of Down's syndrome. *Exp Neurol*, **161**, 647–663.

Gulesserian, T., Engidawork, E., Fountoulakis, M., Lubec, G. (2001) Antioxidant proteins in foetal brain: superoxide dismutase-1 protein is not overexpressed in foetal Down syndrome. *J Neural Transm*, **61** Suppl., 71–84.

Hattori, M., Fujiyama, A., Taylor, T. D., Watanabe, H., Yada, T., Park, H. S., et al. (2000) The DNA sequence of human chromosome 21. *Nature*, **405**, 311–319.

Hauser-Cram, P., Warfield, M. E., Shonkoff, J. P., Krauss, M. W., Sayer, A., Upshurr, C. C. (2001) Children with disabilities: a longitudinal sudy of child development and parent well-being. *Monogr Soc Res Child Dev*, **66**, 1–114.

Hook, E. B. (1981) Unbalanced Robertsonian translocations associated with Down's syndrome or Patau's syndrome: chromosome subtype, proportion inherited, mutation rates, and sex ratio. *Hum Genet*, **59**, 235–239.

Jenkins, E. C., Velinov, M. T. (2001) Down syndrome and the human genome. *Down Syndrome Quarterly*, **6**, 1–12.

Jernigan, T. L., Bellugi, U., Sowell, E., Doherty, S., Hesselink, J. R. (1993) Cerebral morphologic distinction between Williams and Down syndromes. *Arch Neurol*, **50**, 186–191.

Jervis, G. (1948) Early senile dementia in Mongolian idiocy. *Am J Psychiatry*, **105**, 102–106.

Kahlem, P., Sultan, M., Herwig, R., Steinfath, M., Balzereit, D., Eppens, B., et al. (2004) Transcript level alterations reflect gene dosage effects across multiple tissues in a mouse model of Down syndrome. *Genome Res*, **14**, 1258–1267.

Kida, E., Choi-Miura, N.-H., Wisniewski, K. E. (1995) Deposition of apolipoprotein E and J in senile plaques is topographically determined in both Alzheimer's disease and Down's syndrome brain. *Brain Res*, **685**, 211–216.

Kim, S. H., Yoo, B. C., Broers, J. L., Vcairns, N., Lubec, G. (2000) Neuroendocrine specific protein c, a marker of neuronal differentiation, is reduced in brain of patients with Down syndrome and Alzheimer's disease. *Biochem Biophys Res Commun*, **276**, 329–334.

Kish, S., Karlinsky, H., Becker, L., Gilbert, J., Rebbetoy, M., Chang, J., et al. (1989) Down syndrome patients begin life with normal levels of brain cholinergic markers. *J Neurochem*, **52**, 1183–1187.

Korenberg, J. R., Chen, X. N., Schipper, R., Sun, Z., Gonsky, R., Gerwehr, S. et al. (1994) Down syndrome phenotypes; the consequences of chromosomal imbalance. *Proc Natl Acad Sci USA*, **91**, 4997–5001.

Lejeune, J., Gautier, M., Turpin, R. (1959) Etudes des chromosomes somatique de neuf enfants mongoliens. *CR Acad Sci (Paris)*, **240**, 1026–1027.

Lyle, R., Gehrig, C., Neergaard-Henrichsen, C., Deutsch, S., Antonarakis, S. E. (2004) Gene expression from the aneuploid chromosome in trisomy mouse model of Down syndrome. *Genome Res*, **14**, 1268–1274.

Makayev, A. V., Erdenechimeg, L., Mungunsukh, O., Roth, J. J., Enkhmandakh, B., Ruddle, F. H., et al. (2004) GTF21RD2 is located in the Williams-Beuren syndrome critical region 7q11.23 and encodes a protein with two TF-II-I-like helix-loop-helix repeats. *Proc Natl Acad Sci USA*, **101**, 11052–11057.

Mao, R., Zielke, C. L., Zielke, H. R., Pevsner, J. (2003) Global up-regulation of chromosome 21 gene expression in the developing Down syndrome brain. *Genomics*, **81**, 457–467.

Marin-Padilla, M. (1972) Structural abnormalities of the cerebral cortex in human chromosomal aberrations: a Golgi study. *Brain Res*, **44**, 625–629.

Marin-Padilla, M. (1976) Pyramidal cell abnormalities in the mortor cortex of a child with Down's syndrome. *J Comp Neurol*, **167**, 63–81.

Mollgaard, K., Diamond, M. C., Bennett, E. L., Rosenzweig, M. R., Lindner, B. (1971) Quantitative synaptic changes with differential experience in rat brain. *Int J Neurosci*, **2**, 113–128.

Molliver, M. E., Kostovic, I., Vanderloos, H (1973) The development of synapses in cerebral cortex of the human fetus. *Brain Res*, **50**, 403–407.

Oppermann, M., Cols, N., Nyman, T., Helin, J., Saarinen, J., Byman, I., et al. (2000) Identification of foetal brain proteins by two-dimensional gel electrophoresis and mass spectrometry comparison of samples from individuals with or without chromosome 21 trisomy. *Eur J Biochem*, **267**, 4713–4719.

Peterson, A., Patil, N., Robins, C., Wang, J., Cox, D. R., Myers, R. M. (1994) A transcript map of the Down syndrome critical region of chromosome 21. *Hum Mol Genet*, **3**, 1735–1742.

Petit, T. L., LeBoutillier, J. C., Alfano, D. P., Becker, L. E. (1984) Synaptic development in the human fetus: a morphometric analysis of normal and Down's syndrome neocortex. *Exp Neurol*, **83**, 13–23.

Peyrl, A., Weitzdoerfer, R., Gulesserian, T., Fountoulakis, M., Lubec, G. (2002) Aberrant expression of signalling-related proteins 14-3-3 gamma and RACK1 in foetal Down syndrome brain (trisomy 21). *Electrophoresis*, **23**, 152–157.

Pinter, J. D., Eliez, S., Schmitt, J. E., Capone, G. T., Reiss, A. L. (2001) Neuroanatomy of Down's syndrome: a high-resolution MRI study. *Am J Psychiatry*, **158**, 1659–1665.

Pritchard, M. A., Kola, I. (1999) The 'gene dosage effect' hypothesis versus 'the amplified developmental instability' hypothesis in Down syndrome. *J Neural Transm Suppl*, **57**, 293–304.

Purpura, D. P. (1975) Normal and aberrant neuronal development in the cerebral cortex of human fetus and young infants. In N. A., Buchwald, M. A. B. Brazier (eds) *Brain Mechanisms in Mental Retardation*. New York: Academic, pp 141–169.

Rampon, C., Tang, Y. P., Goodhouse, J., Shimizu, E., Kyin, M., Tsien, J. Z. (2000) Enrichment induces structural changes and recovery from nonspacial memory deficits in CA1 NMDAR1-knockout mice. *Nat Neurosci*, **3**, 238–244.

Reeves, R. H., Irving, N. G., Moran, T. H., Wohn, A., Kitt, C., Sisodia, S. S., et al. (1995) A mouse model for Down syndrome exhibits learning and behaviour deficits. *Nat Genet*, **11**, 177–84.

Roizen, N. J., Patterson, D. (2003) Down's syndrome. *Lancet*, **361**, 1281–1289.

Ross, M., Galaburda, A., Kemper, T. (1984) Down's syndrome: is there a decreased population of neurons? *Neurology*, **34**: 909–916.

Schmahmann, J. D., Sherman, J. C. (1998) The cerebellar cognitive affective syndrome. *Brain*, **121**(4), 561–579.

Schmidt-Sidor, B., Wisniewski, K. E., Shepard, T. H., Sersen, E. A. (1990) Brain growth in Down syndrome subjects 15 to 22 weeks of gestational age and birth to 60 months. *Clin Neuropathol*, **9**, 181–190.

Shah, G. N., Bonapace, G., Hu, P. Y., Strisciuglio, P., Sly, W. S. (2004) Carbonic anhydrase II deficiency syndrome (osteopetrosis with renal tubular acidosis and brain calcification): novel mutations in CA2 identified by direct sequencing expand the opportunity for genotype-phenotype correlation. *Hum Mutat*, **24**, 272.

Shapiro, B. L. (1983) Downs syndrome-a disruption of homeostasis. *Am J Med Genet*, **14**, 241–269.

Shapiro, B. L. (1999) The Down syndrome critical region. *J Neural Transm Suppl*, **57**, 41–60.

Shin, J.-H., Gulessarian, T., Weitzdoerfer, R., Fountoulakis, M., Lubec, G. (2004) Derangement of hypothetical proteins in foetal Down's syndrome brain. *Neurochem Res*, **29**, 1307–1316.

Sigman, M., Ruskin, E., Arbeile, S. Corona, R., Dissanayake, C., Espinosa, M., et al. (1999) Continuity and change in the social competence of children with autism, Down syndrome, and developmental delays. *Mon Soc Res Child Dev*, **64**, 1–114.

Takashima, S., Becker, L. E., Amostrong, D. L., Chen, T. (1981) Abnormal neuronal development in the visual cortex in human fetus and infant with Down syndrome. *Brain Res*, **225**, 1–21.

Takashima, S., Fida, K., Mito, T., Arima, M. (1994) Dendritic and histochemical development and aging in patients with Down syndrome. *J Intellect Disabil Res*, **38**, 265–273.

Unterberger, U., Lubec, G., Dierssen, M., Stoltenburg-Didinger, G., Farreras, J. C., Budka, H. (2003) The cerebral cortex in foetal Down syndrome. *J Neural Transm Suppl*, **67**, 159–163.

Venter, J. C., Adams, M. D., Myers, E. W., Li, P. W., Mural, R. J., Sutton, G. G., et al. (2001) The sequence of the human genome. *Science*, **291**, 1304–1351.

Vercauteren, F. G. G., Bergeron, J. J. M., Vandesande, F., Arckens, L., Quirion, R. (2004) Proteomic approaches in brain research and neuropharmacology. *Eur J Pharmacol*, **500**, 385–398.

Vukšić, M., Petanjek, Z., Rasin, M. R., Kostovic, I. (2002) Perinatal growth of prefrontal layer III pyramids in Down syndrome. *Pediatr Neurol*, **27**, 36–38.

Weitzdoerfer, R., Dierssen, M., Fountoulakis, M., Lubec, G. (2001) Foetal life in Down syndrome starts with normal neuronal density but impaired dendritic spines and synaptosomal structure. *J Neural Transm Suppl*, **61**, 59–70.

Wisniewski, K. E. (1990) Down syndrome children often have brain with maturation delay, retardation of growth and cortical dysgenesis. *Am J Med Genet Suppl*, **7**, 274–281.

Wisniewski, K. E., French, J. H., Rosen, J. F., Kozlowski, P. B., Tenner, M., Wisniewski, H. M. (1982) Basal ganglia calcification (BGC) in Down's syndrome (DS)-another manifestation of premature aging. *Ann NY Acad Sci*, **396**, 179–189.

Wisniewski, K. E., Howe, J., Williams, D. G., Wisniewski, H. M. (1978) Precocious aging and dementia in patients with Down's syndrome. *Biol Psychiatry*, **13**, 619–627.

Wisniewski, K. E., Kida, E. (1994) Abnormal neurogenesis and synaptogenesis in Down syndrome brain. *Dev Brain Dysfunct*, **7**, 289–301.

Wisniewski, K. E., Laure-Kamionowska, M., Connell, F., Wen, G. Y. (1986) Neuronal density and synaptogenesis in the postnatal stage of brain maturation in Down syndrome. In C. J. Epstein (ed.) *The Neurobiology of Down Syndrome*. New York NY: Raven Press, pp. 29–45.

Wisniewski, K. E., Laure-Kamionowska, M., Wisniewski, H. M. (1984) Evidence of arrest of neurogenesis and synaptogenesis in brains of patients with Down's syndrome. *N Engl J Med*, **311**, 1187–1188.

Wisniewski, K. E., Schmidt-Sidor, B. (1989) Postnatal delay of myelin formation in brains from Down syndrome infants and children. *Clin Neuropathol*, **8**, 55–62.

Wisniewski, K., Wisniewski, H., Wen, G. (1985) Occurrence of neuropathological changes and dementia of Alzheimer's disease in Down's syndrome. *Ann Neurol*, **17**, 278–282.

Yang, Q., Rasmussen, S. A., Friedman, J. M. (2002) Mortality associated with Down's syndrome in the USA from 1983 to 1997: a population-based study. *Lancet*, **359**, 1019–1025.

Yates, C. M., Simpson, J., Gordon, A., Maloney, A. F. J., Allison, Y., Ritchie, I. M., et al. (1983) Catecholamines and cholinergic enzymes in pre-senile and senile Alzheimer-type dementia and Down's syndrome. *Brain Res*, **280**, 119–126.

Yoo, B. C., Fountoulakis, M., Dierssen, M., Lubec, G. (2001) Expression patterns of cheperone proteins in cerebral cortex of the fetus with Down syndrome, dysregulation of T complex proteins. *J Neural Transm Suppl*, **61**, 321–334.

3 Ageing and Susceptibility to Alzheimer's Disease in Down Syndrome

DAVID PATTERSON

Eleanor Roosevelt Institute, University of Denver, USA

SUMMARY

A relationship between Down syndrome (DS), premature ageing, and Alzheimer's disease (AD) has been observed for many years. Persons with DS invariably develop the neuropathology associated with AD and often develop clinical dementia as well. Recent studies on the molecular events surrounding the pathology of AD and DS strengthen the specificity of this relationship. It appears that oxidative stress, possibly caused by abnormal mitochondrial energy generation and folate metabolism, early endosome abnormalities, abnormalities in APP metabolism and loss of functional cholinergic neurons occur in individuals with DS as in individuals without DS who develop AD. Robust mouse models exist for both DS and AD and study of these has in general confirmed and extended findings with humans. Therapeutic interventions are being undertaken for AD and, to a more limited extent, for DS. Thus, the molecular specificity of the link between DS and AD appears to be robust. Future experiments should allow ever more refined attempts to ameliorate the cognitive decline associated with these conditions.

DOWN SYNDROME AND ALZHEIMER'S DISEASE

One of the most consistent features of DS is its relationship to AD. Evidence for the neuropathological association of DS and AD was first published in English in 1948 (Jervis 1948). Every individual with DS due to full trisomy 21 develops the neuropathology seen in AD. No other syndrome shares this feature with DS. Currently, the most widely accepted hypothesis is that the appearance of amyloid plaques in DS is due to the presence on chromosome 21 of the gene encoding the amyloid precursor protein (APP) leading to

Down Syndrome: Neurobehavioural Specificity. Edited by JA Rondal and J Perera.
© 2006 John Wiley & Sons Ltd.

overexpression of APP and hence overproduction of the Abeta protein, which is the major component of amyloid plaques. One individual with DS who did not develop amyloid plaques was a 78-year-old woman with partial trisomy 21 who had no clinical signs of dementia and on autopsy had no plaques and tangles and was found not to be trisomic for the APP gene (Prasher et al. 1998), an observation consistent with this hypothesis.

A number of investigators hypothesise that trisomy of additional genes on chromosome 21, for example cytosolic superoxide dismutase (SOD1), the S100beta protein, or BACE2, may also contribute to the occurrence of both the neuropathology and the increased risk of AD seen in individuals with DS (Lott & Head 2005). An important question is whether the cognitive decline seen in older individuals with DS parallels the decline seen in individuals in the typical population that develop AD. A recent study suggests that this is indeed so, strengthening the relationship of AD and DS (Nelson et al. 2005).

DOWN SYNDROME AND PRECOCIOUS AGEING

It is less certain whether individuals with DS age more rapidly than chromosomally typical individuals. Historically, Fraser & Mitchell (1876) reported observing 'precipitated senility' in persons with DS in 1876, only 10 years after John Langdon Down described the syndrome (Down 1866) and 30 years prior to the description of AD by Alois Alzheimer (Alzheimer et al. 1907). This issue is complicated by the difficulty in ascertaining how many individuals with DS actually develop AD and how many undergo cognitive decline for other reasons. Until recently, the natural history of DS in adults was difficult to define for at least three reasons. First, the life expectancy of persons with DS was considerably shorter than that of the chromosomally typical population. Second, institutionalisation of large numbers of individuals with DS may have masked the natural history of DS in persons more integrated into society. Third, it can be difficult to assess cognitive decline in a cognitively impaired individual. Currently, many individuals with DS will live at least into their 50s (Yang et al. 2002) and many are not institutionalised. Better methods for assessing cognitive decline have been developed.

Martin (1978) concluded that DS could be considered a 'segmental progeriod syndrome', meaning that persons with DS show many signs associated with ageing in addition to AD. Similarly, Wisniewski et al. (1978) examined 50 persons with DS and concluded that they showed signs of precocious ageing. Various investigators have reported evidence for premature ageing of numerous biological systems in persons with DS, including cognition (Das & Mishra 1995; Fromage & Anglade 2002) the auditory system (Buchanan et al. 1990), the skin (Brugge et al. 1993), brain structure as assessed by MRI (Roth et al. 1996; Sadowski et al. 1999; Teipel et al. 2004), the immune system (Park et al. 2000) and the olfactory system (Nijjar & Murphy 2002). Additionally, it has been reported that persons with DS show an earlier appearance of various biomarkers associated with ageing (Jovanovic et al. 1998; Nakamura & Tanaka 1998; Odetti et al. 1998; Praticò et al. 2000).

Clinically, physicians with extensive experience with persons with DS hypothesise that there is an underlying accelerated ageing in persons with DS (Chicoine et al. 1998; Lott & Head 2005) and that the early and more frequent appearance of AD in persons with DS is simply a feature of more rapid ageing. Interestingly, some features of ageing seem less common in persons with DS. For example, there appears to be a considerably reduced incidence of atherosclerosis and of many solid tumours in persons with DS (Hasle 2001; Lott & Head 2005). These issues require further study to help define the specificity of the occurrence of AD in DS and to determine whether accelerated ageing is indeed a specific, common feature of DS.

METABOLIC CHANGES IN AD, DS AND AGEING

If there is specificity in DS involving premature ageing and AD then one would expect that common mechanisms might play a role in these features. One possibility is metabolic alteration. There are many genes on chromosome 21 that are important for metabolic systems, including oxidative stress due to reactive oxygen species (ROS) and mitochondrial energy metabolism (MT/ROS), transulfuration/one-carbon (TS-1C) metabolism, and cholesterol metabolism that have been hypothesised to play a role in DS, AD, and in ageing itself. Therefore, an examination of the possible similarities in changes in MT/ROS and TS-1C metabolism may help determine whether similar metabolic perturbations occur in DS, AD, and perhaps ageing itself.

MITOCHONDRIA, OXIDATIVE STRESS, DS, AD AND AGEING

One of the dominant theories of ageing is that oxygen (and other) free radicals, or reactive oxygen species (ROS) cause damage to cellular molecules, including DNA, RNA, protein, and lipids and that these accumulate with age leading to malfunctioning of various cell processes. Reactive oxygen species are produced as an inevitable consequence of metabolism and it is estimated that up to 2% of oxygen used for intermediary metabolism is converted to ROS (Floyd & Hensley 2002). The mitochondria, the sites of oxidative phosphorylation and energy generation, produce the vast majority of ROS in mammals (Wallace 2001). The brain is thought to be particularly sensitive to ROS-induced damage because:

- the brain generates and uses about 20% of the energy in a human
- the neurons in the brain are nonreproducing and therefore damage to neurons may be particularly harmful
- the brain contains a large amount of unsaturated fatty acids, which are sensitive to ROS-induced damage (Floyd & Hensley 2002)

Transgenic mice overexpressing catalase targeted to mitochondria have extended lifespans and appear to have an extended period of health as well (Schriner et al. 2005). This result strongly supports the ROS theory of ageing and provides compelling evidence that mitochondria are the source of the ROS that are important in the ageing process (Schriner et al. 2005). Moreover, this result lends support to the concept that ameliorating oxidative stress, if done properly, could ameliorate effects of ageing, AD and perhaps DS.

Oxidative stress is considered by some investigators to be one of the earliest events in AD pathogenesis in the typical population and in persons with DS (Nunomura et al. 2000; Smith et al. 2005). In support of this hypothesis, many investigators have reported increased oxidative stress in AD and in DS. Often, this is accompanied by, and possibly caused by, dysfunctional mitochondria. Busciglio et al. (2002) reported that mitochondrial function and ROS metabolism are altered in neurons and astrocytes cultured from foetuses with DS and that this alteration is associated with altered APP metabolism. This implies that altered oxidative stress may play a role in abnormal brain development in individuals with DS as well as in the neurodegeneration seen later in life. Importantly, elevated levels of isoprostanes (8, $12\text{-}iso\text{-}iPF_{2alpha}$), markers of lipid peroxidation, are elevated in the brains of individuals with DS and also in the brains of individuals with AD (Praticò et al. 2000; Irizarry & Hyman 2003; Yao et al. 2003). The levels of isoprostanes are also elevated in the urine of persons with DS and the levels increase with age (Praticò et al. 2000). The increase in isoprostanes in brains of persons with AD appears to be most striking in the brain regions most highly affected in AD and is not present in other forms of neurodegenerative disease like frontotemporal dementia (Irizarry & Hyman 2003; Yao et al. 2003).

Amyloid precursor protein metabolism has been linked specifically to ROS metabolism. The metabolism of Abeta itself can produce oxidative stress (Nelson & Alkon 2005). Moreover, Abeta has been found to cause aberrant mitochondrial metabolism through binding to a mitochondrial alcohol dehydrogenase (ABAD) that inhibits its activity (Lustbader et al. 2004; Takuma et al. 2005). This interaction has been hypothesised to directly contribute to oxidative stress in AD. Moreover, oxidation of Abeta itself has been hypothesised to be an early event in amyloid plaque biogenesis and perhaps in Abeta pathogenesis (Head et al. 2001). Thus, it appears that there may be an intimate association between APP metabolism associated with AD and DS and abnormal oxidative stress at a fundamental biochemical level. It is important to understand the role of oxidative stress and its relationship to Abeta metabolism because this may lead to new therapeutic approaches to AD and perhaps eventually to DS.

Interestingly, at least 17 genes involved in energy and ROS metabolism, and potentially in APP metabolism, are located on chromosome 21. These are:

- mitochondrial ribosomal protein L39
- ATP synthase F0 coupling factor 6
- NF-E2 related factor (NRF2)
- Bach1
- amyloid precursor protein (APP)
- cytosolic superoxide dismutase (SOD1)
- phosphoribosylgycineamide transformylase (GART)
- NADPH:quinone reductase-like (CRYZL1)
- ATP synthase OSCP subunit
- mitochondrial ribosomal protein S6
- calcipressin 1 (ADAPT78)
- carbonyl reductase 1 (CBR1)
- carbonyl reductase 3 (CBR3)
- thioredoxin-like protein (SH3BGR)
- mitochondrial NADH:oxidoreductase 10 kDa subunit (NDUFV3)
- cystathionine beta synthase (CBS)
- C21orf2 mitochondrial protein

Six of these genes encode mitochondrial proteins. Two of these, ATP synthase F0 subunit 6 and ATP synthase OSCP subunit, comprise part of the stalk of ATP synthase, and thus play important roles in the final step of mitochondrial ATP synthesis (Aggeler et al. 2002). NDUFV3 is a subunit of the catalytic component of oxidative phosphorylation Complex I (de Coo et al. 1997). If these proteins are overexpressed in individuals with DS this could perturb the stoichiometry of these complexes and interfere with their function, potentially leading to oxidative stress.

ONE-CARBON AND FOLIC ACID METABOLISM

Other metabolic systems may be perturbed in AD and DS. One of the most widely studied is the tightly interrelated TS/1-C metabolic system. A simplified representation of this pathway is shown in Figure 3.1. Cystathionine beta synthase (CBS), the gene for which is on chromosome 21, occupies a key position in this metabolic system, linking the folate cycle, the methionine cycle, transulfuration reactions, and the production of the antioxidant glutathione, the major small molecule antioxidant in mammalian brain. At least seven genes important for TS-1C metabolism are present on chromosome 21

- NF-E2 related factor (NRF2)
- putative N6-DNA methyltransferase
- phosphoribosylycineamide transformylase (GART)
- cystathionine beta synthase (CBS)

- DNA methyltransferase 3-like (DNMT3L)
- reduced folate carrier (REFC, SLC19A1)
- formiminotetrahydrofolate cyclodeaminase (FTCD)
- protein arginine N-methyltransferase 1 like-1 (HRMT1L1)

At least three of these are also important for MT/ROS metabolism.

Possible Relationships of Alterations in TS-1C Metabolism, Ageing and AD

Many studies have been published examining the possible role of folate, vitamins B_{12} and B_6, and homocysteine levels in ageing. These studies are by their nature correlative. There is a higher prevalence of folate deficiency in the elderly and it appears that homocysteine levels rise with age (Mattson 2003;

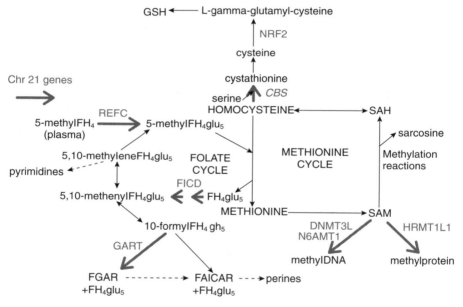

Figure 3.1. A simplified representation of TS/1-C metabolism. Enzymatic steps depicted in grey are encoded on human chromosome 21. Abbreviations are as follows: GSH = glutathione; NRF2 = NF-E2 related factor; CBS = cystathionine beta synthase; SAH = S-adenosylhomocysteine; SAM = S-adenosylmethionine; REFC = reduced folate carrier; FH_4 = tetrahydrofolate; FTCD = formiminotetrahydrofolate cyclodeaminase; GART = phosphoribosylglycineamide transformylase; FGAR = phosphoribosylformylglycineamide; FAICAR = phosphoribosylformylaminoimidazole carboxamide; DNMT3L = DNA methyltransferase 3-like; HRMT1L1 = protein arginine N-methyltransferase 1 like-1; N6AMT1 = putative N6-DNA methyltransferase.

D'Anci & Rosenberg 2004). Elevated homocysteine levels are associated with increased risk of cardiovascular disease and potentially with increased risk of AD and other neurodegenerative disorders (Kado et al. 2005).

Homocysteine arises from dietary methionine, and has two major metabolic fates: one is to be remethylated to methionine and the other is to be converted to cystathionine by the enzyme CBS. Thus, CBS plays a key role in regulating the levels of this important molecule. Folate deficiency leads to elevated homocysteine levels, and folate supplementation can lower homocysteine levels. Recent studies provide correlative evidence for an association between low folate levels and cognitive function and decline in elderly individuals. Low folate may precede the onset of AD (Quadri et al. 2004; Kado et al. 2005). In a study of more severely affected AD patients, a correlation between low folate and cerebral atrophy in individuals with AD was observed (Snowdon et al. 2000). These relationships require much more study.

Possible Relationships of Alterations in TS-1C Metabolism and DS

Possible metabolic abnormalities in DS have been hypothesised for decades. These hypotheses have led to attempts to normalise such abnormalities with various dietary supplements, drugs and other approaches. A recent analysis of published studies on the effects of supplements and drugs on cognitive function in persons with DS found no evidence for benefit with any known treatment (Salman 2002). However, it was also concluded that because of the small numbers of individuals involved and 'the overall unsatisfactory quality of the trials, an effect cannot be excluded at this point' (Salman 2002). Two of the major targets for metabolic intervention are oxidative stress and folate metabolism. The impetus for further study of folate metabolism increased with reports that polymorphisms of some enzymes involved in folate metabolism were associated with increased risk of the birth of a child with DS. This issue remains quite controversial with some studies finding evidence in support of the original data and others being unable to replicate the findings. A recent invited comment (James 2004) summarises the status of these complex studies. It seems likely that it may be a combination of metabolic state and genotype that is important. Moreover, if the effect on folate metabolism is upon non-disjunction during female meiosis, any effects of folate metabolism may have been important in the grandmother of the child with DS (James 2004). A study that may be relevant to this issue is the report of an increase in frequency of births of children with DS in families in which a neural tube defect has occurred and vice-versa (Barkai et al. 2003). Considering the known ability of folate supplementation to decrease the incidence of neural tube defects, this finding can be interpreted as suggesting a relationship between neural tube defects, DS, and folate metabolism.

The presence of CBS on chromosome 21 would suggest that if CBS is over-expressed according to gene dosage in persons with DS then homocysteine levels would be low. Even this is somewhat controversial. Some studies indeed find lowered homocysteine levels (Pogribna et al. 2001), while others do not (Fillon-Emery et al. 2004). A recent publication (Guéant et al. 2005) reported that relatively high homocysteine levels are associated with low IQ in persons with DS. In this report, levels of homocysteine tended to be slightly lower in persons with DS.

The Connection between Folate, CBS and Oxidative Stress

In vitro studies using cell culture models and *in vivo* studies using rodents show that folate deficiency leading to elevated homocysteine can cause oxidative stress and that supplementation with folate can alleviate oxidative stress induced by chemicals (Ho et al. 2003; Huang et al. 2004). Interestingly, transcription of the CBS gene itself may be sensitive to ROS concentrations (Mosharov et al. 2000; MacLean et al. 2002). This appears to allow enhancement of production of cysteine and glutathione, the major small molecule antioxidant in mammalian cells, in response to oxidative stress (Mosharov et al. 2000; Vitvitsky et al. 2004). The transcription factor Nrf2, the gene for one subunit of which is located on chromosome 21, regulates the synthesis of glutathione. In rats and canines, glutathione levels decrease with age (Head et al. 2002). Recent evidence suggests that the mechanism for this reduction may be a decline in transcriptional activity of Nrf2 (Suh et al. 2004). It is not currently known whether age-related decline in transcription of Nrf2 occurs in DS, AD, or human ageing. In any case, these and other experiments may suggest Nrf2 activity as a possible target to ameliorate neurodegeneration (Calkins et al. 2005).

MOUSE MODELS OF AD AND DS

Much, but not all, of the work described above on humans is correlative. For ethical as well as scientific reasons, many experiments to understand the alterations in cognition and behaviour associated with DS and AD cannot be done on humans. Dietary studies have their own particular challenges. It is difficult to control diet sufficiently over long periods of time in large numbers of humans and to take into account the interplays between many metabolic systems (Niculescu & Zeisel 2002; Salman et al. 2002). Time constraints make some experimental interventions impractical in humans. Of course, the validity of animal models depends on how well they mimic the human situation. Some elegant studies on canines that develop amyloid plaques as they age and on ageing rats indicate that oxidative stress may play a role in the loss of learning and memory associated with ageing and that the learning and memory losses can be ameliorated by dietary supplementation with antioxidants and enhancers of mitochondrial function (Liu et al. 2002; Milgram et al. 2004). However no models of DS exist in these species. Fortunately, good mouse models for DS and AD are available. Therefore, it is possible to determine with considerable accuracy whether these animal models provide evidence for a specific relationship between DS and AD.

The Ts65Dn mouse was first described in 1990 (Davisson et al. 1990). It was produced to serve as a mouse model of DS. It is the most robust mouse model of DS thus far available and shows many features also seen as part of the phenotype of DS. (See Davisson & Costa 1999 and Patterson & Costa 2005 for a description of some of the features of these mice.) Ts65Dn mice do not show accumulation of amyloid plaques and neurofibrillary tangles. However, recent evidence indicates that older Ts65Dn mice have elevated levels of APP and Abeta (Hunter et al. 2003, 2004; Seo & Isacson 2005). Ts65Dn mice show significant deficits in the Morris Water Maze that suggest alterations in hippocampal function (Stasko & Costa 2004 and references therein).

Hippocampal function is inordinately affected in DS (Pennington et al. 2003) and is a hallmark of AD (Selkoe 2002). There is a striking loss of learning and memory with age and a concomitant loss of cholinergic phenotype reminiscent of what is seen in AD and elderly individuals with DS in Ts65Dn mice (Holtzman et al. 1996; Granholm et al. 2000; Hyde & Crnic 2001). The mice lose, in an age-dependent manner, functional basal forebrain cholinergic neurons as assessed by immunostaining with anti-TrkA, Chat, or p75 antibodies (Holtzman et al. 1996; Hyde & Crnic 2001; Granholm et al. 2000). This is similar to what is observed in persons with AD and older persons with DS (Davies et al. 1987; Mann et al. 1987; Mufson et al. 2000). Synaptic structural abnormalities in Ts65Dn mice appear similar to those seen in DS as well (Belichenko et al. 2004). Interestingly, the loss does not appear to be due entirely to the death of cells but due to their lack of expression of cholinergic markers (Cooper et al. 2001).

Cooper et al. (2001) examined nerve growth factor (NGF) processing in the brains of young and old Ts65Dn mice. They found that NGF levels were essentially normal in the hippocampus of old Ts65Dn and that the basal forebrain cholinergic neurons (BFCN) could bind and internalise NGF normally but that it could not be transported to the cell bodies. Thus, there is a deficit in retrograde transport of NGF. If NGF was supplied directly to the BFCN cell bodies, the immunostaining was restored.

Nerve growth factor is a neurotrophic factor that is critical for neuronal survival and function. Therapy with NGF for AD has been tried but side-effects were unacceptable (Tuszynski et al. 2005). In a phase I clinical trial, NGF-producing autologous fibroblasts were injected into the forebrains of several individuals with mild AD. These cells colonised the region of the

brain near the injection site and produced NGF. Of potentially great significance, in this small study there appeared to be a significant slowing of the
progression of AD as assessed by two cognitive tests commonly used to assess
cognitive decline in persons with AD and the treatment was well tolerated
(Tuszynski et al. 2005). The improvement was more significant than that
observed with the most common treatments for AD.

One of the earliest detectable abnormalities in the brains of individuals
with AD or DS appears to be an alteration in early endosome function well
before the appearance of plaques (reviewed in Nixon 2005). These abnormalities include the localisation of Abeta in the abnormal endosomes and are
essentially indistinguishable in AD and DS. Moreover, essentially identical
abnormalities are observed in the Ts65Dn mice. APP must play a role in these
abnormalities because when Ts65Dn mice, which are trisomic for the APP
gene, are bred with mice in which one copy of APP is inactivated, some of
the offspring are typical Ts65Dn mice except that they have only two copies
of the mouse APP gene. These mice do not show the early endosome abnormality. Moreover, mice trisomic for the APP gene alone do not show the
abnormality. Therefore, APP is necessary but not sufficient for the early
endosome abnormality.

It is thought that early endosomes function in the uptake of NGF at synapses and retrograde transport to BCFN cell bodies, thus playing a critical
role in NGF signalling (Howe & Mobley 2005). This is consistent with the
finding that axonal transport is aberrant in mouse models of AD (Stokin et
al. 2005). Indeed, many of the features observed in Ts65Dn mice are also
observed in numerous transgenic mouse models of AD.

It is unlikely that NGF treatment will ameliorate completely the features
of AD, and its effect in DS is not known, although the experiments with
Ts65Dn mice are encouraging. Importantly, other agents are being tested in
the Ts65Dn mice for efficacy in alleviating the learning and memory decline
seen in these animals. Of particular note, oestrogen seems to be beneficial in
female, but apparently not male, Ts65Dn mice (Granholm et al. 2002). Of
more general interest, treatment with minocycline can ameliorate the loss of
functional cholinergic neurons and also the learning and memory difficulties
seen in the Ts65Dn mice (Hunter et al. 2004). The mechanism of action of
minocycline in this system is not understood, however, it is known to have
anti-inflammatory properties and also appears to protect against cell death
by preserving mitochondrial function (Wang et al. 2004a).

SYNAPTIC DYSFUNCTION – WHERE IT MAY ALL
COME TOGETHER

It appears that AD, the loss of cognitive ability in elderly individuals with DS
and the loss of learning and memory in mouse models all have many specific

features in common at the biochemical and molecular level. An attractive hypothesis with much evidence to support it is that the crucial event is synaptic dysfunction and that this begins prior to the appearance of plaques and tangles. It appears to be related to alterations in APP metabolism, however, and recent evidence suggests that excessive Abeta protein can suppress synaptic function and that synaptic function can modulate Abeta metabolism (Kamenetz et al. 2003). Synapses require high levels of energy, a fact consistent with a role for mitochondrial dysfunction in synapse dysfunction. Clearly, retrograde transport of early endosomes requires energy as well, so it seems that a part of the pathology of AD and DS may also involve aberrant mitochondrial function and energy generation. Again, evidence suggests that Abeta can directly and negatively affect mitochondrial function (Lustbader et al. 2004; Takuma et al. 2005). This could have the added consequence of causing elevated oxidative stress that is part of these conditions. Clearly, elevated oxidative stress can affect synaptic function as well. In this regard, folate deficiency and elevated homocysteine levels appear to sensitise neurons to Abeta toxicity (Kruman et al. 2002; Mattson & Shea 2003).

These specific common features of AD and DS imply that there will be numerous possible treatments that may work for both conditions. It seems likely that a combination of approaches, for example, correction of aberrant NGF trafficking, targeted treatments to improve mitochondrial function and ways to minimise oxidative stress, including normalisation of folate and one-carbon metabolism, may be required to ameliorate the cognitive disabilities associated with AD and with DS.

FUTURE DIRECTIONS

None of the mouse models currently available are complete models of DS, and additional mouse models of AD are continually becoming available. With regard to the Ts65Dn mice, an approach that holds significant promise is the breeding of these mice with mice bearing single active copies of individual genes or sets of genes trisomic in the Ts65Dn mice to help define more precisely the roles of trisomy of individual genes in DS and also the roles of other genes on chromosome 21 in AD. This may extend the specific nature of the deficits seen in DS and AD.

Ts65Dn mice are not trisomic for the genes on human chromosome 21 that are on mouse chromosomes 17 and 10. For example, they are not trisomic for at least five genes that play a role in one-carbon and folate metabolism. Thus, they are not optimal for studying the role perturbation of this pathway may play in DS. They are not trisomic for genes important for cholesterol metabolism, notably the ABCG1 gene, the product of which is likely to play an important role in cholesterol trafficking (Wang et al. 2004b). This is significant because aberrant cholesterol metabolism has been hypothesised to exist in DS and to play a role in AD pathogenesis as well (Lott & Head 2005). Many signalling pathways have been hypothesised to play roles in both AD and DS. In several cases, genes on human chromosome 21 participate in these pathways but so do genes on other chromosomes. This means that systems biology and computational biology methods will be important to understand how the complex interconnections of these biological pathways interact (Gardiner et al. 2004; Patterson & Costa 2005).

Another feature of DS and of ageing and AD that needs to be addressed is the wide variability in all these conditions. Identification of particular combinations of gene polymorphisms that influence this variability would seem to be a fruitful approach. Indeed, this genetic variability may well be a confounding factor in attempts to define specificity in DS. It may be that specific gene polymorphism patterns will be associated with specific variations in phenotype. These sets of polymorphisms may define, among other things, how individuals respond to their environment and to various therapeutic approaches. Evidence for this phenomenon is already accumulating in analysis of the TS-1C metabolic pathway, in which a variety of polymorphisms in several of the enzymes in the pathway are known to influence the precise functioning of the pathway and to have health consequences. Fortunately, the multidisciplinary tools are now at hand to approach all these issues. In this way it may be possible to define much more precisely the specificity of the phenotypes of DS in genetic and molecular terms and to relate specific genetic profiles more precisely with the variations seen in DS and indeed in AD and ageing.

REFERENCES

Aggeler, R., Coons, J., Taylor, S. W., Ghosh, S. S., Garcia, J. J., Capaldi, R. A., et al. (2002) A functionally active human $F_1 F_o$ ATPase can be purified by immunocapture from heart tissue and fibroblast cell lines. *J Biol Chem*, **277**, 33905–33912.

Alzheimer, A., Stelzmann, R. A., Schnitzlein, H. N., Murtagh, F. R. (1995) An English translation of Alzheimer's 1907 paper, 'Ober eine eigenartige Erkankung der Hirnrinde'. *Clin Anat*, **8**, 429–431.

Barkai, G., Arbuzova, S., Berkenstadt, M., Heifetz, S., Cuckle, H. (2003) Frequency of Down's syndrome and neural-tube defects in the same family. *Lancet*, **361**, 1331–1335.

Belichenko, P. V., Masliah, E., Kleschevnikov, A. M., Villar, A. J., Epstein, C. J., Salehi, A., Mobley, W. C. (2004) Synaptic structural abnormalities in the Ts65Dn mouse model of Down syndrome. *J Comp Neurol*, **480**, 281–298.

Brugge, K. L, Grove, G. L., Cloptin, P., Grove, M. J., Piacquadio, D. J. (1993) evidence for accelerated skin wrinkling among developmentally delayed individuals with Down's syndrome. *Mechanisms of Aging and Development*, **70**, 213–225.

Buchanan, L. H. (1990) Early onset of presbyacusis in Down syndrome. *Scandinavian Audiology*, **19**, 103–110.

Busciglio, J., Pelsman, A., Wong, C., Pigino, G., Yuan, M., Mori, H., et al. (2002) Altered metabolism of the Amyloid β precursor protein is associated with mitochondrial dysfunction in Down's syndrome. *Neuron*, **33**, 677–688.

Calkins, M. J., Jakel, R. J., Johnson, D. A., Chan, K., Kan Y. W., Johnson J. A. (2005) Protection from mitochondrial complex II inhibition in vitro and in vivo by Nrf2-mediated transcription. *Proc Natl Acad Sci Unit States Am*, **102**, 244–249.

Chicoine, B., McGuire, D., Rubin, S. S. (1998) Adults with Down syndrome: Specialty clinic perspectives. In M. P. Janicki, A. J. Dalton (eds) *Dementia, Aging, and Intellectual Disabilities: A Handbook*. New York: Brunner/Mazel, pp. 278–293.

Cooper, J. D., Salehi, A., Delcroix, J-D., Howe, C. L., Belichenko, P. V., Chua-Couzens, J., et al. (2001) Failed retrograde transport of NGF in a mouse model of Down's syndrome: Reversal of cholinergic neurodegenerative phenotypes following NGF infusion. *Proc Natl Acad Sci Unit States Am*, **98**, 10439–10444.

D'Anci, K. E., Rosenberg, I. H. (2004) Folate and brain function in the elderly. *Curr Opin Clin Nutr Metab Care*, **7**, 659–664.

Das, J. P., Mishra, R. K. (1995) Assessment of cognitive decline qassociated with aging: a comparison of individuals with Down syndrome and other etiologies. *Res Dev Disabil*, **16**, 11–25.

Davies, C. A., Mann, D. M., Sumpter, P. Q., Yates, P. O. (1987) A quantitative morphometric analysis of the neuronal and synaptic content of the frontal and temporal cortex in patients with Alzheimer's disease. *J Neurol Sci*, **78**, 151–164.

Davisson, M. T., Schmidt, C., Akeson, E. C. (1990) In Patterson, D., Epstein C. (eds) *Molecular Genetics of Chromosome 21 and Down Syndrome*. New York: Wiley-Liss, pp. 263–280.

Davisson, M. T., Costa, A. C. S. (1999) Mouse models of Down syndrome. In B. Popko (ed.) *Advances in Neurochemistry. Volume 9. Mouse Models of Human Genetic Neurological Disease*. New York: Plenum Publishing Corp., pp. 297–327.

De Coo, R. F., Buddiger, P., Smeets, H. J., Van Oost, B. A. (1997) Molecular cloning and characterization of the human mitochondrial NADH:oxidoreductase 10-kDa gene (NDUFV3). *Genomics*, **45**, 434–437.

Down, J. H. L. (1866) Observations on an ethnic classification of idiots. *Lond Hosp Rep*, **3**, 259–262. Reprinted in *Ment Retard*, **33**, 54–56, 1995.

Fillon-Emery, N., Chango, A., Mircher, C., Barbé, F., Bléhaut, H., Herbeth, B., et al. (2004) Homocysteine concentrations in adults with trisomy 21: effect of B vitamins and genetic polymorphisms. *Am J Clin Nutr*, **80**, 1551–1557.

Floyd, R. A., Hensley, K. (2002) Oxidative stress in brain aging. Implications for therapeutics of neurodegenerative diseases. *Neurobiology of Aging*, **23**, 795–807.

Fraser, M., Mitchell, A. (1876) Kalmyc idiocy. *J Ment Sci*, **22**, 169–179.

Fromage, B., Anglade, P. (2002) The aging of Down's syndrome subjects. *Encephale*, **28**, 212–216.

Gardiner, K., Davisson, M. T., Crnic, L. S. (2004) Building protein interaction maps for Down's syndrome. *Briefings in Functional Genomics and Proteomics*, **3**, 142–156.

Granholm, A.-C. E., Ford, K. A., Hyde, L. A., Bimonte, H. A., Hunter, C. L., Nelson, M., et al. (2002) Estrogen restores cognition and cholinergic phenotype in an animal model of Down syndrome. *Physiology Behavior*, **77**, 371–385.

Granholm, A.-C. E., Sanders, L. A., Crnic, L. S. (2000) Loss of cholinergic phenotype in basal forebrain coincides with cognitive decline in a mouse model of Down's syndrome. *Exp Neurol*, **161**, 647–663.

Guéant, J.-L., Anello, G., Bosco, P., Guéant-Rodriguez, R.-M., Romano, A., Barone, C., et al. (2005) Homocysteine and related genetic polymorphisms in Down's syndrome IQ. *Journal of Neurology, Neurosurgery, and Psychiatry*, available at http://jnnp.bmjjournals.com, 706–709.

Hasle, H. (2001) Pattern of malignant disorders in individuals with Down's syndrome. *Lancet Oncology*, **2**, 429–436.

Head, E., Garzon-Rodriguez, W., Johnson, J. K., Lott, I. T., Cotman, C. W., Glabe, C. (2001) Oxidation of Aβ and plaque biogenesis in Alzheimer's disease and Down syndrome. *Neurobiol Dis*, **8**, 792–806.

Head, E., Liu, J., Hagen, T. M., Muggenberg, B. A., Milgrams, N. W., Ames, B. N., et al. (2002) Oxidative damage increases with age in a canine model of human brain aging. *J Neurochem*, **82**, 375–381.

Ho, P. I., Ashline, D., Dhitavat, S., Ortiz, D., Collins, S. C., Shea, T. B., et al. (2003) Folate deprivation induces neurodegeneration: roles of oxidative stress and increased homocysteine. *Neurobiol Dis*, **14**, 32–42.

Holtzman, D. M., Santucci, D., Kilbridge, J., Chua-Couzens, J., Fontana, D. J., Daniels, S. E., et al. (1996) Developmental abnormalities and age-related neurodegeneration in a mouse model of Down syndrome. *Proc Natl Acad Sci Unit States Am*, **93**, 13333–13338.

Howe, C. L., Mobley, W. C. (2005) Long-distance retrograde neurotrophic signaling. *Curr Opin Neurobiol*, **15**, 40–48.

Huang, R.-F. S., Yaong, H.-C., Chen, S.-C., Lu, Y.-F. (2004) In vitro folate supplementation alleviates oxidative stress, mitochondria-associated death signaling and apoptosis induced by 7-ketocholesterol. *Br J Nutr*, **92**, 887–894.

Hunter, C. L., Bachman, D., Granholm, A.-C. (2004) Minocycline prevents cholinergic loss in a mouse model of Down's syndrome. *Ann Neurol*, **56**, 675–688.

Hunter, C. L., Isacson, O., Nelson, M., Bimonte-Nelson, H., Seo, H., Lin, L., et al. (2003) Regional alterations in amyloid precursor protein and nerve growth factor across age in a mouse model of Down's syndrome. *Neurosci Res*, **45**, 437–445.

Hyde, L. A., Crnic, L. S. (2001) Age-related deficits in context discrimination learning in Ts65Dn mice that model Down syndrome and Alzheimer's disease. *Behav Neurosci*, **15**, 1239–1246.

Irizarry, M. C., Hyman, B. T. (2003) Brain Isoprostanes. A marker of lipid peroxidation and oxidative stress in AD. *Neurobiol*, **61**, 436–437.

James, S. J. (2004) Maternal metabolic phenotype and risk of Down syndrome: beyond genetics. *Am J Med Genet*, **127A**, 1–4.

Jervis, G. A. (1948) Early senile dementia in mongoloid idiocy. *Am J Psychiatr*, **105**, 102–106.

Jovanovic, S. V., Clements, D, MacLeod, K. (1998) Biomarkers of oxidative stress are significantly elevated in Down syndrome. *Free Radic Biol Medic*, **25**, 1044–1048.

Kado, D. M., Karlamangla, A. S., Huang, M.-H., Troen, A., Rowe, J. W., Selhub, J., et al. (2005) Homocysteine versus the vitamins folate, B_6, and B_{12} as predictors of cognitive function and decline in older high-functioning adults: MacArthur Studies of Successful Aging. *Am J Med*, **118**, 161–167.

Kamenetz, F., Tomita, T., Hsieh, H., Seabrook, G., Borchelt, D., Iwatsubo, T., Sisodia, S., Malinow, R. (2003) APP processing and synaptic function. *Neuron*, **37**, 925–937.

Kruman, I. I., Kumaravel, T. S., Lohani, A., Pederson, W. A., Cutler, R. G., Kruman, Y., et al. (2002) Folic acid deficiency and homocysteine impair DNA repair in hippocampal neurons and sensitize them to amyloid toxicity in experimental models of Alzheimer's disease. *J Neurosci*, **22**, 1752–1762.

Liu, J., Head, E., Gharib, A. M., Yuan, W., Ingersoll, R. T., Hagen, T. M., et al. (2002) Memory loss in old rats is associated with brain mitochondrial decay and RNA/DNA oxidation: partial reversal by feeding acetyl-L-carnitine and/or R-α-lipoic acid. *Proc Natl Acad Sci Unit States Am*, **99**, 2356–2361.

Lott, I. T., Head, E. (2005) Alzheimer disease and Down syndrome: factors in pathogenesis. *Neurobiol Aging*, **26**, 383–389.

Lustbader, J. W., Cirilli, M., Lin, C., Xu, H. W., Takuma, K., Wang, N., et al. (2004) ABAD directly links Aβ to mitochondrial toxicity in Alzheimer's disease. *Science*, **304**, 448–452.

MacLean, K. N., Janošík, M., Kraus, E., Kožich, V., Allen, R. H., Raab, B. K., et al. (2002) Cystathionine β-synthase is coordinately regulated with proliferation through a redox sensitive mechanism in cultured human cells and Saccharomyces cerevisiae. *J Cell Physiol*, **192**, 81–92.

Mann, D. M., Yates, P. O., Marcyniuk, B., Ravindra, C. R. (1987) Loss of neurons from cortical and subcortical areas in Down's syndrome patients at middle age. Quantitative comparisons with younger Down's patients and patients with Alzheimer's disease. *J Neurol Sci*, **80**, 79–89.

Martin, G. M. (1978) Genetic syndrome in man with potential relevance to the pathobiology of aging. In D. Bergsma, D. E. Harrison (eds) *Genetic Effects on Aging, Birth Defects: Original Article Series*, Volume XIV(1). New York: Alan R. Liss, pp. 5–39.

Mattson, M. P. (2003) Gene-diet interactions in brain aging and neurodegenerative disorders. *Ann Intern Med*, **139**, 441–444.

Mattson, M. P, Shea, T. B. (2003) Folate and homocysteine metabolism in neural plasticity and neurodegenerative disorders. *Trends Neurosci*, **26**, 137–146.

Milgram, N. W., Head, E., Zicker, S. C., Ikeda-Douglas, C., Murphey, H., Muggenberg, B. A., et al. (2004) Long-term treatment with antioxidants and a program of behavioral enrichment reduces age-dependent impairment in discrimination and reversal learning in beagle dogs. *Experimental Gerontology*, **39**, 753–765.

Mosharov, E., Cranford, M. R., Banerjee, R. (2000) The quantitatively important relationship between homocysteine metabolism and glutathione synthesis by the transsulfuration pathway and its regulation by redox changes. *Biochemistry*, **39**, 13005–13011.

Mufson, E. J., Ma, S. Y., Cochran, E. J., Bennett, D. A., Beckett, L. A., Jaffar, S., et al. (2000) Loss of nucleus basalis neurons containing trkA immunoreactivity in individuals with mild cognitive impairment and early Alzheimer's disease. *J Comp Neurol*, **427**, 19–30.

Nakamura, E., Tanaka, S. (1998) Biological ages of adult men and women with Down's syndrome and its changes with aging. *Mech Ageing Dev*, **105**, 89–103.

Nelson, L., Johnson, J. K., Freeman, M., Lott, I., Groot, J., Chang, M., et al. (2005) Learning and memory as a function of age in Down syndrome: a study using animal-based tasks. *Progr Neuro Psychopharmacol Biol Psychiatr*, **29**, 443–453.

Nelson, T. J., Alkon, D. L. (2005) Oxidation of cholesterol by amyloid precursor protein and beta-amyloid peptide. *J Biol Chem*, **280**, 7377–7387.

Niculescu, M. D, Zeisel, S. H. (2002) Diet, methyl donors and DNA methylation: inter-actions between dietary folate, methionine and choline. *J Nutr*, **132**, 2333S–2335S.

Nijjar, R. K. Murphy, C. (2002) Olfactory impairment increases as a function of age in persons with Down syndrome. *Neurobiol Aging*, **23**, 65–73.

Nixon, R. A. (2005) Endosome function and dysfunction in Alzheimer's disease and other neurodegenerative diseases. *Neurobiol Aging*, **26**, 373–382.

Nunomura, A., Perry, G., Pappolla, M. A., Friedland, R. P., Hirai, K., Chiba, S., Smith, M. A. (2000) Neuronal oxidative stress precedes Amyloid-β deposition in Down syndrome. *Journal of Neuropathology and Experimental Neurology*, **39**, 1011–1017.

Odetti, P., Angelini, G., Dapino, D., Zaccheo, D., Garibaldi, S., Dagna-Bricarelli, F., et al. (1998) Early glycoxidation damage in brains from Down's syndrome. *Biochem Biophys Res Comm*, **243**, 840–851.

Park, E., Alberti, J., Mehta, P., Dalton, A., Sersen, E., Levis, G. S. (2000) Partial impairment of immune functions in peripheral blood leukocytes from aged men with Down's syndrome. *Clin Immunol*, **95**, 62–69.

Patterson, D., Costa, A. C. S. (2005) Down syndrome and genetics – a case of linked histories. *Nature Reviews/Genetics*, **6**, 137–147.

Pennington, B. F., Moon, J., Edgin, J., Stedron, J. Nadel, L. (2003) The neuropsych-ology of Down syndrome: evidence for hippocampal dysfunction. *Child Dev*, **74**, 85–93.

Pogribna, M., Melnyk, S., Pogribny, I., Chango, A., Yi, P., James, S. J. (2001) Homo-cysteine metabolism in children with Down syndrome: in vitro modulation. *Am J Hum Genet*, **69**, 88–95.

Prasher, V. P., Farrer, M. J., Kessling, A. M., Fisher, E. M. C., West, R. J., Barber, P. C. et al. (1998) Molecular mapping of Alzheimer-type dementia in Down's syndrome. *Ann Neurol*, **43**, 380–383.

Praticò, D., Iuliano, L, Amerio, G., Tang, L. X., Rokach, J., Sabatino, G., et al. (2000) Down's syndrome is associated with increased 8,12-iso-iPF$_{2\alpha}$-VI levels: Evidence for enhanced lipid peroxidation in vivo. *Ann Neurol*, **48**, 795, 798.

Quadri, P., Fragiacomo, C., Pezzati, R., Zunda, E., Forloni, G., Tettamanti, M., et al. (2004) Homocysteine, folate, and vitamin B-12 in mild cognitive impairment, Alzheimer disease, and vascular dementia. *Am J Clin Nutr*, **80**, 114–122.

Roth, G. M., Sun, B., Greensite, F. S., Lott, I. T., Dietrich, R. B. (1996) Premature aging in persons with Down syndrome: MR findings. *Am J Neuroradiol*, **17**, 1283–1289.

Sadowski, M., Wisniewski, H. M., Tarnawski, M., Kozlowski, P. B., Lach, B., Wegiel, J. (1999) Entorhinal cortex of aged subjects with Down's syndrome shows severe neuronal loss caused by neurofibrillary pathology. *Acta Neuropath*, **97**, 156–164.

Salman, M. S. (2002) Systematic review of the effect of therapeutice dietary supple-ments and drugs on cognitive function in subjects with Down syndrome. *Eur J Paediatr Neurol*, **6**, 213–219.

Schriner, S. E., Linford, N. J., Martin, G. M., Tareuting, P., Ogburn, C. E., Emond, M., et al. (2005) Extension of murine life span by overexpression of catalse targeted to mitochondria. *Science*, **308**, 1909–1911.

Selkoe, D. J. (2002) Alzheimer's disease is a synaptic failure. *Science*, **298**, 789–791.

Seo, Y., Isacson, O. (2005) Abnormal APP, cholinergic and cognitive function in Ts65Dn Down's model mice. *Experimental Neurobiology*, **193**, 469–480.

Smith, M. A., Nunomura, A., Lee, H.-G., Zhu, X., Moreira, P. J., Avila, J., et al. (2005) Chronological primacy of oxidative stress in Alzheimer disease. *Neurobiol Aging,* **26**, 579–580.

Snowdon, D. A., Tully C. L., Smith, C. D., Riley, K. P., Markesbery, W. R. (2000) Serum folate and the severity of atrophy of the neocortex in Alzheimer disease: findings from the Nun study. *Am J Clin Nutr,* **71**, 993–998.

Stasko, M. R., Costa, A. C. (2004) Experimental parameters affecting the Morris water maze performance of a mouse model of Down syndrome. *Behav Brain Res,* **154**, 1–17.

Stokin, G. B., Lillo, C., Falzone, T. L., Brusch, R. G., Rockenstein, E., Mount, S. L., et al. (2005) Axonopathy and transport deficits early in the pathogenesis of Alzheimer's disease. *Science,* **307**, 1282–1288.

Suh, J. H., Shenvi, S. V., Dixon, B. M., Liu, H., Jaiswal, A. K., Liu, R.-M., et al. (2004) Decline in transcriptional activity of Nrf2 causes age-related loss of glutathione synthesis, which is reversible with lipoic acid. *Proc Natl Acad Sci Unit States Am,* **101**, 3381–3397.

Takuma, K., Yao, J., Huang, J., Xu, H., Chen, X., Luddy, J., et al. (2005) ABAD enhances Aβ-induced cell stress via mitochondrial dysfunction. *FASEB Journal,* **19**, 597–598.

Teipel, S. J., Alexander, G. E., Schapiro, M. B., Möller, H.-J., Rapoport, S. I., Hampel, H. (2004) Age-related cortical grey matter reductions in non-demented Down's syndrome adults determined by MRI with voxel-based morphometry. *Brain,* **127**, 811–824.

Tuszynski, M. H., Thal, L., Pay, M., Salmon, D. P., Bakay, R., Patel, P., et al. (2005) A phase 1 clinical trial of nerve growth factor gene therapy for Alzheimer disease. *Nat Med,* **11**, 551–555.

Vitvitsky, V., Dayal, S., Stabler, S., Zhou, Y., Wang, H., Lentz, S. R., et al. (2004) Perturbations in homocysteine-linked redox homeostasis in a murine model for hyperhomocysteinemia. *American Journal of Physiology-Regulatory Integrative and Comparative Physiology,* **287**, R39–R46.

Wallace, D. C. (2001) Mitochondrial defects in neurodegenerative disease. *Mental Retardation and Developmental Disabilities: Research Reviews,* **7**, 158–166.

Wang, J., Wei, Q., Wang, C.-Y., Hill, W. D., Hess, D. C. Dong, Z. (2004a) Minocycline up-regulates Bcl-2 and protects against cell death in mitochondria. *J Biol Chem,* **279**, 19948–19954.

Wang, N., Lan, D., Chen, W., Matsuura, F., Tall, A. R. (2004b) ATP-binding cassette transporters G1 and G4 mediate cellular cholesterol efflux to high-density lipoproteins. *Proc Natl Acad Sci Unit States Am,* **101**, 9774–9779.

Wisniewski, K., Howe, J., Williams, D. G., Wisnieski, H. M. (1978) Precocious aging and dementia in patients with Down's syndrome. *Biol Psychiat,* **13**, 619–627.

Yang, Q., Rasmussen, S. A., Friedman, J. M. (2002) Mortality associated with Down's syndrome in the USA from 1983 to 1997: a population-based study. *The Lancet,* **359**, 1019–1025.

Yao, Y., Zhukareva, V., Sung, S., Clark, C. M., Rokach, J., Lee, et al. (2003) Enhanced brain levels of 8-12-iso-iPF$_{2\alpha}$-VI differentiate AD from frontotemporal dementia. *Neurology,* **61**, 475–478.

4 Down Syndrome Specificity in Health Issues

ALBERTO RASORE QUARTINO
Ospedale Galliera, Genova, Italy

SUMMARY

Down Syndrome (DS) is caused by the trisomy of chromosome 21, whose entire DNA sequence is now complete and is predicted to contain about 300 genes. Phenotypic expression of DS is well known but whether it could be considered specific is a controversial question. Trisomy 21 is the single condition causing the sequentially phenotypic features and clinical consequences of DS, most of which also occur in other situations. Careful overview of the health issues present in DS and in other genetic syndromes enables the observer to ascertain to what degree these syndromes can reasonably be considered specific. The pattern of phenotypic features pertaining to each genetic syndrome makes them specific. This review discusses some of the most informative features, pointing out distinctive aspects in clinical manifestations of DS. It concludes that many items show specific representations in DS – from increased frequency (congenital heart defects (CHD), autoimmune disorders, leukaemia) to reduced frequency (bronchial asthma, solid cancer), from different expression (CHD, outcome in AML, sensitivity to leukaemia therapies) to uniqueness (transient leukaemia – TL). Further studies are necessary to identify more effectively gene products and their effects on the phenotype of DS.

INTRODUCTION

Down syndrome is the most common autosomal disorder in humans and is caused by the trisomy of chromosome 21. Its prevalence ranges from 1 : 700 to 1 : 1000 live births. Very recently the chromosome 21 DNA sequence was completed and is predicted to contain about 300 genes (Capone 2001). Despite this achievement, little is known about the mechanisms whereby the phenotypic characteristics of the syndrome are produced. Gene dosage imbalance is actually considered responsible either directly or through complex gene interactions (Antonarakis et al. 2004).

Down Syndrome: Neurobehavioural Specificity. Edited by JA Rondal and J Perera.
© 2006 John Wiley & Sons Ltd.

Many of the phenotypic traits show large individual variation but neuro-motor dysfunction, cognitive and language impairment are observed in virtually all individuals. In addition, for any given phenotype there is considerable variability in expression. Congenital malformations occur with increased incidence: CHD and congenital malformations of the gastrointestinal tract are the most frequent. Congenital laxity of connective tissue is common. People with DS are prone to develop autoimmune disease (for example, hypothyroidism, coeliac disease, diabetes mellitus, thrombocytopenia). Growth retardation is almost invariable. Early ageing is also constant.

Epidemiology has distinctive aspects: DS is the most frequent chromosomal aneuploidy with cognitive impairment in humans; the abortion rate is also very high: spontaneous foetal loss occurs in more than 60% of pregnancies; survival has increased through the years and individuals with DS can now reach 60 years and over.

The main characteristics of DS are:

• trisomy of chromosome 21 (300 genes)
• phenotypic features
• cognitive and language impairment
• neuromotor dysfunction
• growth reduction
• congenital heart disease (50%)
• immune dysfunction and autoimmune disorders
• early ageing/pathological ageing
• reduced survival

Whether or not there is a specificity in DS health issues is controversial. Many elements have to be considered. First, the chromosomal anomaly, trisomy 21, which by itself is the condition causing sequentially phenotypic features and clinical manifestations, most of which do indeed occur in other syndromes. A careful overview of the health issues in DS and in other genetic syndromes enables the observer to ascertain, for each, differences in the manner of presentation, in frequency, in severity and in clinical consequences that make the word 'specificity' sound reasonable. The pattern of phenotypic features pertaining to each genetic syndrome makes them specific.

This review discusses some of the most interesting and informative features and points out specific aspects of clinical manifestations of DS.

CONGENITAL MALFORMATIONS

HEART DEFECTS

Congenital heart defects (CHD) occur in over 40% of individuals with DS compared to a figure of 0.5% to 1% in infants with normal chromosomes.

The specificity of chromosome 21 for endocardial cushion defects is illustrated by the finding that 70% of all endocardial defects are associated with DS; the majority of endocardial cushion defects found in the population as a whole are those associated with DS. Moreover, in infants with trisomy 21 mosaicism there is a lower incidence of CHD (30%) and these are less severe (Marino and DeZorzi 1993).

Frequently found CHD are atrioventricular canal defect (36% to 47%), ventricular septal defect (26% to 33%), atrial septal defect and tetralogy of Fallot.

The process of heart formation requires the fine integration of several molecular and morphogenetic events and must involve the action of a large number of genes. The high incidence of CHD in DS strongly suggests that genes mapping to chromosome 21 could be involved in heart morphogenesis and that their abnormal expression in trisomy 21 could disturb heart development, although genes located on other chromosomes could also be responsible for CHD.

Recently, the CRELD1 gene (cysteine rich with EGF domains), mapping to chromosome 3p25, was recognised as the first genetic risk factor for atrioventricular septal defect (AVSD) (Robinson et al. 2003). Mutations of this gene increase susceptibility to AVSD but are not sufficient to cause the defect, suggesting that AVSD is multigenic (Maslen 2004).

It is noteworthy that congenital heart defects in DS are less severe and more predictable than in other infants. As a consequence, surgical results can sometimes be better than those obtained in patients with the same heart malformation but without chromosome abnormalities (Marino et al. 2004).

In adults with DS a high prevalence (up to 70%) of mitral valve prolapse and aortic regurgitation was recognised. It is possible that both these defects are the consequence of the congenital laxity of connective tissue.

Intersyndromic comparison for CHD shows interesting differences: Turner syndrome (45, X) is associated with severe narrowing of whole aortic arch (Hyett et al. 1997) and partial anomalous pulmonary venous drainage (Mazzanti & Cacciari 1998). In a recent survey of 117 individuals, Volkl et al. (2005) observed that 30% had cardiovascular anomalies, mainly left sided and associated with aortic structure defects. Aortic malformations were most frequent (72.8%), represented by coarctation of the aorta and bicuspid aortic valve.

Klinefelter syndrome (47, XXY), on the other hand, is generally not associated with congenital heart defects (Simpson et al. 2003).

Trisomy 18 has cardiac defects in almost all individuals (Hyett et al. 1995). The commonest cardiac lesions are ventricular septal defects and/or polyvalvular abnormalities.

In trisomy 13, congenital cardiac lesions are less frequent and among them there are atrioventricular or ventricular septal defects, valvular abnormalities and narrowing of the isthmus or truncus arteriosus (Hyett et al. 1997).

OTHER CONGENITAL MALFORMATIONS

Gastrointestinal malformations in DS are more frequent than in non-Down infants: duodenal stenosis (4% to 7%) represents nearly half of all congenital duodenal stenoses. Hirschprung disease is present in 3% to 4% of newborns with DS, versus 0.02% of other infants.

Muscular and orthopaedic anomalies are well known in DS. Muscular hypotonia and joint hyperlaxity are almost constant. They are important causes of walking problems, even of severe static troubles such as scoliosis and cyphosis. Prevention through active life and sport activities is effective.

The clinical significance of atlanto axial instability received particular attention in recent years, although it was known as an entity not specifically related to DS. In fact it has been described as the result of trauma (37%), in rheumatoid arthritis (29%), as a result of prior surgery (21%) and as a result of congenital abnormalities (12%) (Haid et al. 2001). It was also described in Marfan syndrome (Herzka et al. 2000) and following infectious processes of the upper respiratory tract (Griesel syndrome) (Wurm et al. 2004). Its prevalence is elevated in DS: 10% to 15% (Pueschel & Schola 1987), 15% to 20% according to Menezes & Ryken (1992). It is usually asymptomatic, but an increased risk of dislocation exists, with subsequent severe neurological complications ((Menezes & Ryken 1992). The value of various diagnostic methods is controversial (Selby et al. 1991). Children at risk should not be allowed to practise dangerous sport activities. For symptomatic cases surgical stabilisation with different techniques (vertebral fusion or transarticular screw fixation) has proved successful (Aicardi 1992, Toussaint et al. 2003).

CANCER

The occurrence of cancer is unique in DS, with a high risk of leukaemia in children and a reduced risk of solid tumours in all age groups, except for retinoblastoma, ovarian cancer and testicular cancer (Hasle et al. 2000; Goldacre et al. 2004). In children with DS there is a 20-fold increased risk of developing leukaemia (Goldacre et al. 2004). Leukaemia is nevertheless a very uncommon disease even in DS.

The developments in research generally define the pivotal role played by chromosome 21 both in childhood acute lymphoblastic leukemia (ALL) and acute myeloblastic leukemia (AML). Children with DS account for approximately 3% of children with ALL and 5% to 8% of children with AML. Moreover, a particularly high risk (500-fold higher risk) exists for one type of AML, acute megakaryoblastic leukaemia (AMKL, M7AML): 20% of leukaemias of DS are AMKL (Zipursky et al. 1987; Zipursky 2003). There is also an almost fourfold higher incidence of AML to ALL in children with DS and the incidence of AML is highly skewed towards the younger age with only rare cases appearing beyond age 5 years.

One of the most singular expressions of DS is the disorder known as transient myeloproliferative disorder (TMD) or transient leukaemia (TL), which is characterised by the accumulation of immature megakaryocites in peripheral blood, in liver and bone marrow (Zipursky 2003). It is typically seen in newborns and has a high incidence of spontaneous remissions. It occurs in approximately 10% of newborns and might not be recognised in mild cases without a careful observation of peripheral blood smears (Taub & Ravindranath 2002). Not more than 10% of cases are routinely diagnosed (Bradbury 2005). Although largely clinically silent, in some cases it is life threatening. In severe cases, the infant may be born with hydrops foetalis and may show evidence of multi-organ failure, pulmonary hypertension and respiratory failure (Smrceck et al. 2001; Hoskote et al. 2002). Neonatal and prenatal mortality may range from 11% to 55%. Up to 30% of those who achieve spontaneous remission will subsequently develop AMKL within the first 4 years of life (Massey 2005).

Pathogenesis of TMD/TL and of AMKL has recently been connected with acquired mutations of the GATA1 gene (mapping to chromosome X), which have been detected almost exclusively in DS patients affected with these forms. The transcription factor GATA1 is needed for normal growth and maturation of erythroid cells and megakaryocytes. The observed mutations resulted in a premature translation termination, eliminating the GATA1 activation domain encoded by exon 2 (Orkin, 2000). These mutations prevent synthesis of full-length GATA1, but not synthesis of a shorter variant GATA1s, whose expression could confer a proliferative advantage to the mutant GATA1 clones, so favouring their expansion and survival. The mutations can occur prenatally and, as they can exist in the absence of leukaemia, they can be an early step in an otherwise multistep process of leukemogenesis (Taub et al. 2004).

It is current opinion that TL is a disorder of foetal hepatic hemopoiesis. Its spontaneous resolution could be related to its physiological reduction and disappearance at birth, substituted by medullary hemopoiesis (Crispino 2005). The finding of an identical GATA1 mutation in sequential samples collected from a patient during TL and subsequent AMKL would confirm the same origin of both forms (Hitzler et al. 2003). A model of malignant transformation to AMKL in DS is proposed, in which GATA1 mutations are an early event and AMKL arises from latent TL clones following initial apparent remission (Hitzler & Zipursky 2005).

While in DS an increased susceptibility to acute leukaemia is observed, on the other end there is an enhanced sensitivity to chemotherapy (Ravindranath 2003). Epidemiological data have shown that the outcome of ALL in children with DS is equivalent or somewhat inferior to non-Down children, possibly due to the increased infection rate or to less intensive salvage therapy offered to children with DS in relapse. The toxicity of methotrexate in these patients is well known. A reduced clearance of the drug and an increased intracellular transport are among the causes of this toxicity and of the increased sensitivity to therapy.

A surprising observation refers to the extremely high event-free survival (80% to 100%) and lower relapse rates (<15%) in children with DS and AML, in particular AMKL, compared to non-Down children (Taub & Ge 2005). AMKL has a very poor outcome in non-Down children (<25% cure) (Lange et al. 1998). The better outcome of AML in children with DS is actually multifactorial in origin and can be related to the enhanced sensitivity of DS AML to ARA-C and other anthracyclines. A possible reason appears to be the increased expression of the gene cystathyonine-beta-synthase (CBS, mapping to chromosome 21q22.3) that can act on the ARA-C metabolism (Ge et al. 2003). Somatic mutations of GATA-1 could in turn be able to modify the expression of target genes, altering the metabolism of the same drugs. Another factor could be the increased generation of oxygen radicals for the enhanced expression of the SOD gene (mapping to chromosome 21) and the increased spontaneous apoptosis in multiple cell systems of DS.

It is not clear whether DS patients with particularly severe TL should be treated and how. Repeated courses of low-dose ARA-C have been used effectively in a small number of children (Cominetti et al. 1985; Zipursky 1996). This raises the intriguing possibility that such a treatment may even prevent the subsequent occurrence of AMKL (Ravindranath 2005).

A different pattern of cancer susceptibility is observed in other chromosomal syndromes: the occurrence of mediastinal germ-cell tumour and breast cancer has been repeatedly reported in men with Klinefelter syndrome, whereas the incidence of ALL and other hematologic malignancies does not seem to be increased (Machatschek et al. 2004). In Turner syndrome there is evidence of the occurrence of gonadal tumour from dysgenetic gonads and of nongonadal neoplasia, among which neurogenic tumours show a preponderance in children and young adults (Sivakumaran et al. 1999).

GROWTH RETARDATION

Growth retardation in DS is certainly multifactorial in origin. There is no growth hormone (GH) deficiency although a suboptimal endogenous production due to hypothalamic dysfunction was recorded. Serum deficiency of IGF-I was observed (Sara et al. 1983; Barreca et al. 1994) but not of IGF-II (Annerén et al. 1984).

Short-term GH therapy increased growth velocity and stature in children with DS but growth velocity declined after cessation of treatment. During GH therapy no increase of head volume was observed and there was no effect on mental or motor functions. GH therapy is not recommended in people with DS (Annerén et al. 1999).

IMMUNE DISORDERS

Disorders of the immune system in DS are constant and complex. Classically a substantial increased risk of infectious diseases was demonstrated although at present extended use of vaccinations and of antibiotic therapy has greatly reduced this susceptibility, reaching values similar to those of the normal population.

Many abnormal aspects of immunology have been described in DS.

The thymus is small and has structural anomalies, with lymphoid depletion, poor corticomedullary demarcation and a thin cortex; Hassal corpuscles are increased and thymic humoral factors decreased.

Antibody-mediated immunity is deranged, with an overall increased antibody level.

More severe abnormalities exist in cell-mediated immunity, with altered maturation of T lymphocytes, inverted CD4/CD8 rate. An abnormal number of functionally deficient NK cells was also demonstrated (Ugazio 1981; Nespoli et al. 1993).

Noncontroversial issues in DS immunology include:

- hypoplasia and alterations of the thymic structure with lymphocyte depletion
- elevated antibody levels
- altered maturation of T lymphocytes with CD4/CD8 rate reversal and functional deficiency
- high number of functionally deficient NK cells

Recent investigation has shown that a rare disorder, the autoimmune polyendocrine syndrome type I (APS-I), is caused by a mutation in the AIRE (autoimmune regulator) gene mapping to chromosome 21q22.3 (Meyer & Badenhoop 2002). The high prevalence of autoimmune disease in DS might be due to dysregulation of the AIRE gene. Autoimmune disorders in DS include:

- thyroiditis (15%)
- coeliac disease (6%)
- type I diabetes mellitus (1%)
- idiopathic juvenile arthritis (1%)
- thrombocytopenia
- chronic active hepatitis
- autoimmune polyendocrine syndrome (APS) type 1

Hypothyroidism has an increased incidence in DS.

Persistent primary congenital hypothyroidism affects 0.07% to 1% of newborns with DS, versus 0.015% to 0.020% newborns in the general population. Acquired hypothyroidism is also greatly increased. Reported data range from 3% to 54%, versus values ranging from 0.8% to 1.1% in the normal population.

Thyroid autoantibodies have been detected in 13% to 34% of people with DS. Autoimmune thyroid disease is uncommon in preschool children with DS but it occurs commonly after the age of 8 years (Karlsson et al. 1998). The pathogenesis of thyroid disorders in DS seems to be correlated with a combination of thyroid autoimmunity and progressively thyroid gland hypoplasia.

Unique to DS is a condition characterised by the persistent increase in the concentration of TSH, associated with a normal concentration of thyroxine. Coeliac disease (CD), or gluten intolerance, is an autoimmune gastrointestinal disorder observed with increased frequency in DS. Its prevalence reaches 6%, whereas in the general population it is as low as 0.43%. Moreover, in the general population, silent forms of CD are more frequent than clinically symptomatic forms (8:1) whereas this ratio is reversed in DS (1:4). It can be hypothesised that mechanisms of compensation are present in people without DS so that enteropathy may exist for a long time without symptoms, whereas in DS people these mechanisms are less able to overcome the overt clinical manifestations of CD (Bonamico et al. 2001).

Anti-gliadin antibodies are a weak marker for CD in DS, contrary to what occurs in people with normal chromosomes. Determination of serum antiendomysium antibodies is a more useful screening test in DS. The determination of anti-tissue transglutaminase is the most recent assay. This enzyme plays a key pathogenetic role in CD because it activates the autoimmune process responsible for the disease, through the modification of the gliadin peptides (Dieterich et al. 1998). Since tissue transglutaminase is now known to be the antigen recognised by antiendomisium antibodies, the transglutaminase antibody test is accurate as a screening test for CD in DS (Hoffenberg et al. 2000).

The genetic susceptibility to CD seems associated with the major histocompatibility complex (MHC) encoded within the Class II region of chromosome 6. Until now no support has been provided for genetic linkage of CD to chromosome 21.

We noted a reduced incidence of asthma in a cohort of 551 subjects: only one had mild episodes between 2 and 5 years of age (Forni et al. 1990). This was more recently confirmed in a cohort of 1453 people with DS (Goldacre et al. 2004). We suggested that the immunodeficient state in DS might confer a measure of protection against the development of bronchial asthma. Another possibility is that they may be less predisposed than others to asthma, or that they may have more infections early in life, with reduced antibody production against self antigens.

CHROMOSOME 21

The sequencing of chromosome 21 was a turning point for the understanding of DS. Recent research is beginning to identify the functional components of the chromosome.

Two categories of genes are on chromosome 21. There are dosage-sensitive and non-dosage sensitive genes. Only the first ones have an effect on the phenotype, when present in three copies. The effect on the phenotype could be either direct or indirect. The indirect effect might be due to the interaction with genes or gene products of other chromosomes. Their effect on the phenotype may be allele specific and have a threshold effect.

Finally, triplication of certain conserved functional non-genic sequences (CNG) might contribute to the DS phenotype.

To complicate this very complex picture, the hypothesis of overexpression (1.5-fold) of the genes that are present in three copies has been partially challenged in the partial trisomy mouse model, showing that only a fraction of genes are overexpressed at the theoretical value, while others are not overexpressed or are expressed at levels differing greatly from the expected values (Antonarakis et al. 2004).

All these data highlight the complex regulation of gene expression related to genomic dosage imbalance in DS.

CONCLUSION

As we have seen in this (necessarily incomplete) review, many items show distinctive representations in DS. Features occurring with increased frequency include:

- congenital heart defects
- gastrointestinal malformations
- leukaemia
- autoimmune disorders
- atlantoaxial instability
- muscular hypotonia
- reduced growth
- early ageing

Features occurring with decreased frequency include:

- solid cancer
- asthma

Features occurring with different expression include:

- congenital heart defects
- response of leukemias to therapy
- coeliac disease

Transient leukaemia occurs exclusively in DS.

The complex pattern of clinical manifestations in DS represents a peculiar feature because, although most components can often be found in other conditions, their sum pertains only to trisomy 21.

More precise connections with genomic imbalance of genes mapping either to chromosome 21 or to other chromosomes and a better identification of gene products and their effects on the phenotype are currently under study.

In a general way, each genetic syndrome has its own specificity. From a practical point of view, specific health care protocols and specific treatments (rehabilitative, educational and so on) are already available for the most frequent syndromes. Ongoing research will be able to better define more specific issues in each syndrome, allowing the delineation of still more effective therapeutic and rehabilitative policies.

REFERENCES

Aicardi, J. (1992) *Diseases of the Nervous System in Childhood.* London: McKeith Press.

Annerén, G., Engberg, G., Sara, V. R. (1984) The presence of normal levels of immunoreactive insulin-like growth factor 2 (IGF-2) in patients with Down's syndrome. *Ups J Med Sci*, **89**, 274–278.

Annerén, G., Tuvemo, T., Carlsson-Skwirut, C., Lonnerholm, T., Bang, P., Sara, V. R., Gustafsson, J. (1999) Growth hormone treatment in young children with Down's syndrome: effects on growth and psychomotor development. *Arch Dis Child*, **80**, 334–338.

Antonarakis, S. E., Lyle, R., Dermitzakis, E. T., Reymond, A., Deutsch, S. (2004) Chromosome 21 and Down syndrome: from genomics to pathophysiology. *Nature*, **5**, 725–738.

Barreca, A., Rasore Quartino, A., Acutis, M. S. (1994) Assessment of growth hormone insulin like growth factor-I axis in Down's syndrome. *Journal of Endocrinological Investigation*, **17**, 431–436.

Bonamico, M., Mariani, P., Danesi, H. M., Crisogianni, M., Failla, P., Gemme, G., et al. (2001) Prevalence and clinical picture of celiac disease in italian Down sindrome patients: a multicenter study. *Journal of Pediatric Gastroenterology and Nutrition*, **33**, 139–143.

Bradbury, J. (2005) High leukaemia cure rate in Down's syndrome explained. *The Lancet*, **6**, 134.

Capone, G. T. (2001) Down syndrome: advances in molecular biology and the neurosciences. *J Dev Behav Pediatr*, **22**, 40–59.

Cominetti, M., Rasore-Quartino, A., Acutis, M. S., Vignola, G. (1985) Neonato con sindrome di Down e leucemia mieloide acuta. Difficoltà diagnostiche fra forma maligna e sindrome mieloproliferativa. *Pathologica*, **77**, 625–630.

Crispino, J. D. (2005) GATA1 mutations in Down syndrome: implications for biology and diagnosis of children with transient myeloproliferative disorder and acute megakaryoblastic leukaemia. *Pediatr Blood Cancer*, **44**, 45–44.

Dieterich, W., Laag, E., Schopper, H., Volta, U., Ferguson, O., Gillet, H., et al. (1998) Autoantibodies to tissue transglutaminase as predictors of celiac disease. *Gastroenterology*, **115**, 1317–1321.

Forni, G. L., Rasore Quartino, A., Acutis, M. S., Strigini, P. (1990) Incidence of bronchial asthma in Down syndrome (letter). *J Pediat*, **116**, 487.

Ge, Y., Jensen, T. L., Matherly, L. H., Taub, J. W. (2003) Transcriptional regulation of the cystathionine-beta-synthase gene in Down syndrome and non-Down syndrome megakaryocytic leukaemia cell lines. *Blood*, **101**, 1551–1557.

Goldacre, M. J., Wotton, C. J., Seagroatt, V., Yeates, D. (2004) Cancer and immune related diseases associated with Down's syndrome: a record linkage study. *Arch Dis Child*, **89**, 1014–1017.

Haid, R. W. Jr, Subach, B. R., McLaughlin, M. R., Rodts, G. E. Jr, Wahlig, J. B. Jr (2001) C1-C2 transarticular screw fixation for atlantoaxial instability: a 6-year experience. *Neurosurgery*, **49**, 65–68.

Hasle, H., Clemmensen, I. H., Mikkelsen, M. (2000) Incidence of cancer in individuals with Down syndrome. *Tidsskr Nor Laegeforen*, **120**, 2878–2881.

Herzka, A., Sponseller, P. D., Pyeritz, R. E. (2000) Atlantoaxial rotatory subluxation in patients with Marfan syndrome. A report of three cases. *Spine*, **25**, 524–526.

Hitzler, J. K., Cheung, J., Li, Y., Scherer, S. W., Zipursky, A. (2003) GATA1 mutations in transient leukaemia and acute megakaryoblastic leukaemia of Down syndrome. *Blood*, **101**, 4301–4304.

Hitzler, J. K., Zipursky, A. (2005) Origins of leukaemia in children with Down syndrome. *Nature Reviews*, **5**, 11–20.

Hoffenberg, E. J., Bao, F., Eisenbarth, G. S., Uhlhorn, C., Haas, J. E., Sokol, R. J., et al. (2000) Transglutaminase antibodies in children with a genetic risk for celiac disease. *J Pediatr*, **137**, 356–360.

Hoskote, A., Chessells, J., Pierce, C. (2002) Transient abnormal myelopoiesis (TAM) causing multiple organ failure. *Intensive Care Med*, **28**, 758–762.

Hyett, J. A., Moscoso, G., Nicolaides, K. H. (1995) Cardiac defects in 1st trimester fetuses with trisomy 18. *Fetal Diagn Ther*, **10**, 381–386.

Hyett, J. A., Moscoso, G., Nicolaides, K. H. (1997) Abnormalities of the heart and great arteries in first trimester chromosomally abnormal fetuses. *Am J Med Genet*, **69**, 207–216.

Karlsson, B., Gustafsson, J., Hedow, G., Ivarsson, S. A., Annerén, G. (1998) Thyroid function in children and adolescents with Down syndrome in relation to age, sex, growth velocity and thyroid antibodies. *Arch Dis Childhood*, **79**, 242–245.

Lange, B. J., Kobrinsky, N., Barnard, D. R., Arthur, D. C., Buckley, J. D., Howells, W. B., et al. (1998) Distinctive demography, biology and outcome of acute myeloid leukaemia and myelodysplastic syndrome in children with Down syndrome: Children's Cancer Group Studies 2861 and 2891. *Blood*, **91**, 608–615.

Machatschek, J. N., Schrauder, A., Helm, F., Schrappe, M., Claviez, A. (2004) Acute lymphoblastic leukaemia and Klinefelter syndrome in children: two cases and review of the literature. *Pediatr Hematol Oncol*, **21**, 621–626.

Marino, B., Assenza, G., Mileto, F., Digilio, M. (2004) Down syndrome and congenital heart disease. In J. A. Rondal, A. Rasore-Quartino, S. Soresi (eds) *The Adult with Down Syndrome. A New Challenge for Society.* London: Whurr Publishers, pp. 39–50.

Marino, B., DeZorzi, A. (1993) Congenital heart disease in trisomy 21 mosaicism. *J Pediatr,* **122**, 500–501.

Maslen, C. L. (2004) Molecular genetics of atrioventricular septal defects. *Curr Opin Cardiol,* **19**, 205–210.

Massey, G. V. (2005) Transient leukaemia in newborns with Down syndrome. *Pediatr Blood Cancer,* **44**, 29–32.

Mazzanti, L., Cacciari, E. (1998) Congenital heart disease in patients with Turner's syndrome. Italian Study Group for Turner Syndrome (ISGTS). *J Pediatr,* **133**, 688–692.

Menezes, A. H., Ryken, T. C. (1992) Craniovertebral anomalies in Down's syndrome. *Pediatr Neurosurg,* **18**, 24–33.

Meyer, G., Badenhoop, K. (2002) Autoimmune regulator (AIRE) gene on chromosome 21: implications for autoimmune polyendocrynopathy-candidiasis-ectodermal dystrophy (APECED) any more common manifestation of endocrine autoimmunity. *J Endocrinol Invest,* **25**, 804–811.

Nespoli, L., Burgio, G. R., Ugazio, A.G., Maccario, R. (1993) Immunological features of Down's sindrome: a review. *J Intellect Disabil Res,* **37**, 543–551.

Orkin, S. H. (2000) Diversification of haemopoietic stem cells to specific lineages. *Nat Rev Genet,* **1**, 57–64.

Pueschel, S. M., Schola, F. H. (1987) Atlantoaxial instability in individuals with Down syndrome: epidemiologic, radiographic and clinical studies. *Pediatrics,* **80**, 555, 560.

Ravindranath, Y. (2003) Down syndrome and acute myeloid leukaemia: the paradox of increased risk for leukaemia and heightened sensitivity to chemotherapy. *J Clin Oncol,* **21**, 3385–3387.

Ravindranath, Y. (2005) Down syndrome and leukaemia: new insights into the epidemiology, pathogenesis and treatment (commentary). *Pediatr Blood Cancer,* **44**, 1–7.

Robinson, S. W., Morris, C. D., Goldmuntz, E., Reller, M. D., Jones, M. A., Steiner, R. D., et al. (2003) Missense mutations in CRELD1 are associated with cardiac atrioventricular septal defect. *Am J Hum Genet,* **72**, 1047–1052.

Sara, V. R., Gustavson, K. H., Annerén, G., Hall, K., Wetterberg, L. (1983) Somatomedins in Down's syndrome. *Biol Psychiat,* **18**, 803–811.

Selby, K. A., Newton, R. W., Gupta, S., Hunt, L. (1991) Clinical predictors and radiological reliability in atlantoaxial subluxation in Down's syndrome. *Arch Dis Child,* **66**, 876–878.

Simpson, J. L., De la Cruz, F., Swerdloff, R. S., Samango-Sprouse. C., Skakkebaek, N. E., Graham, J. E., et al. (2003) Klinefelter syndrome: expanding the phenotype and identifying new research directions. *Genet Med,* **5**, 460–468.

Sivakumaran, T. A., Ghose, S., Kumar, H., Singha, U., Kucheria, K. (1999) Nongonadal neoplasia in patients with Turner syndrome. *J. Environ Pathol Toxicol Oncol,* **18**, 339–347.

Smrceck, J. M., Baschat, A. A., Germer, U., Gloeckner-Hofmann, K., Gembruch, U. (2001) Fetal hydrops and hepatosplenomegaly in the second half of pregnancy: a sign of myeloproliferative disorder in fetuses with trisomy 21. *Ultrasound Obstet Gynecol,* **17**, 403–409.

Taub, J. W., Ge, Y. (2005) Down syndrome, drug metabolism and chromosome 21. *Pediatr Blood Cancer*, **44**, 33–39.

Taub, J. W., Mundschau, G., Ge, Y., Poulik, J. M., Qureshi, F., Jensen, T., et al. (2004) Prenatal origin of GATA1 mutations may be an initiating step in the development of megakaryocytic leukaemia in Down syndrome. *Blod*, **104**, 1588–1589.

Taub, J. W., Ravindranath, Y. (2002) Down syndrome and the transient myeloproliferative disorder: why is it transient? *Journal of Pediatric Hematology/Oncology*, **24**, 6–8.

Toussaint, P., Desenclos, C., Peltier, J., LeGars, D. (2003) Transarticular atlanto-axial screw fixaton for treatment of C1-C2 instability. *Neurochirurgie*, **49**, 519–526.

Ugazio, A. G. (1981) Down's syndrome: problems of immunodeficiency. *Hum Genet Suppl*, **2**, 33–39.

Volkl, T. M., Degenhardt, K., Koch, A., Simm, D., Dorr, H. G., Singer, H. (2005) Cardiovascular anomalies in children and young adults with Ullrich-Turner syndrome. The Erlangen experience. *Clin Cardiol*, **28**, 88–92.

Wurm, G., Aichholzer, M., Nussbaumer, K. (2004) Acquired torticollis due to Griesel's syndrome: case report and follow-up of non-traumatic atlantoaxial rotatory subluxation. *Neuropediatrics*, **35**, 134–138.

Zipursky, A. (1996) The treatment of children with megakaryoblastic leukaemia who have Down syndrome. *J Pediatr Hematol Oncol*, **18**, 10–12.

Zipursky, A. (2003) Transient leukaemia – a benign form of leukaemia in newborn infants with trisomy 21. *Br J Haematol*, **120**, 930–938.

Zipursky, A., Peeters, M., Poon, A. (1987) Megakaryoblastic leukaemia and Down's syndrome: a review. *Pediatr Haematol Oncol*, **4**, 211–230.

5 Neuropsychological Aspects of Down Syndrome

LYNN NADEL
University of Arizona, Tucson, USA

SUMMARY

Down syndrome (DS) is the most prevalent cause of mental retardation. In most cases it results from an extra chromosome 21. In the past few decades much has been learned about the neural underpinnings of the cognitive defect observed in this syndrome but complete understanding remains a distant goal. This chapter reviews what is known about brain and cognitive function in DS, looking at data from studies with individuals at all ages. Although there is a general intellectual defect in DS it is clear that neural and cognitive impairments are not observed uniformly across all domains; in DS there is a specific pattern of deficits implicating problems with the hippocampal formation, the prefrontal cortex and perhaps the cerebellum. This highly specific pattern distinguishes DS from other forms of mental retardation such as Williams syndrome (WS), autism, Prader-Willi syndrome and others. Making progress on ameliorating the difficulties faced by individuals with DS will require careful attention to be given to its highly specific nature.

INTRODUCTION

Down syndrome, the most common cause of mental retardation, has a well-known cause – triplication of all or much of chromosome 21. Yet we still do not understand exactly how to characterise the cognitive impairments in DS. This lack of understanding makes it hard to improve the lives of individuals whose development follows an atypical path. In this chapter I will consider cognitive and neuropsychological function in DS in terms of specific features that help differentiate it from other forms mental retardation. This specificity is an important clue to what actually causes the form of retardation observed in DS.

Down Syndrome: Neurobehavioural Specificity. Edited by JA Rondal and J Perera.
© 2006 John Wiley & Sons Ltd.

THE GENERAL DEFECT

Individuals with DS typically fall in the range of mild to moderate retardation, with IQs in the range of 50 to 90. Some individuals with DS fall within the normal range, while others are severely retarded. This variability is itself a significant challenge but is hardly surprising given the nature of the disorder.

In considering the causes of this intellectual impairment one can seek explanations at multiple, not necessarily exclusive, levels. I focus here on two levels: neurobiological and cognitive.

THE NEUROBIOLOGY OF DS

At birth it is often difficult to differentiate the brains of normal and DS individuals. Yet, both post mortem and neuroimaging studies have demonstrated clear differences between these two groups as early as 6 months of age. Where do these differences come from, and what do they amount to?

The brains of individuals with DS are typically smaller than those of age-matched controls, at least after 6 months of age. However, these differences in brain size could be a matter of allometry. This possibility, added to the fact that there is no clear relation between brain size and 'intelligence' in any event, suggests that the mental retardation observed in DS is not simply a result of gross differences in brain size.

Although the brains of DS individuals are smaller overall, some brain areas are disproportionately affected. This differential impact is not predicted by allometry, and presumably offers important clues about how trisomy 21 brings about the mental retardation so characteristic of DS.

Early studies showed that the brain of an individual with DS at or shortly before birth is in many respects indistinguishable from the brain of a normal individual (Brooksbank et al. 1989; Wisniewski & Schmidt-Sidor 1989; Florez et al. 1990; Schmidt-Sidor et al. 1990; Bar-Peled et al. 1991; Pazos et al. 1994). Normal values were reported for brain and skull shape, brain weight, proportion of specific cerebral lobes, size of cerebellum and brain stem, and the emergence of most neurotransmitter systems. There is evidence, however, that some changes begin to emerge as early as 22 weeks gestational age (for example, Schmidt-Sidor et al. 1990; Golden & Hyman 1994; Wisniewski & Kida 1994; Engidawork & Lubec 2003) and it is clear that by the age of 6 months a number of important differences are already obvious. Some of these differences are expressed in terms of the proportion of individuals with DS who show abnormal values, rather than in terms of a uniform abnormality in all instances. This is important as it highlights the variability in this population sharing the genotypic feature of trisomy 21. (It is an open question how individuals with DS compare to typically developing individuals in terms of variability – there are plausible reasons to imagine more variability, less variability, or normal variability. This is an important research question for the future.)

One noticeable difference concerns a postnatal delay in myelination (Wisniewski 1990), global at first but then manifested primarily in nerve tracts that are myelinated especially late in development, such as the fibres linking the frontal and temporal lobes. This delay is observed in about 25% of infants with DS who come to post mortem analysis between the ages of 2 months and 6 years. Delayed myelination has also been observed in a study employing magnetic resonance imaging on a single infant (18 months of age) with DS (Koo et al. 1992). While not underestimating the impact of this myelination delay, it is worth noting that in all cases myelination is within normal range at birth, while in 75% of the cases it is within normal range throughout early development. Becker et al. (1986) showed that dendritic arborisations in visual cortex of individuals with DS were paradoxically greater than normal early in infancy but then considerably less than normal by the age of 2 years. They speculate that the initial overabundance might result from a compensatory response to the absence of adequate synapse formation, but the fact remains that by early childhood there is an impoverishment in neocortex.

Neuropathological differences after 3 to 5 months of age include a shortening of the fronto-occipital length of the brain, which appears to result from a reduction in growth of the frontal lobes, a narrowing of the superior temporal gyrus (observed in about 35% of cases), a diminished size of the brain stem and cerebellum (observed in most cases) and a 20% to 50% reduction in the number of cortical granular neurons (see Crome et al. 1966; Benda 1971; Blackwood & Corsellis 1976). Notwithstanding these differences, the overall picture at birth or shortly thereafter is one of only modest abnormalities, although individuals with DS tend to fall towards the bottom of the normal range (or outside it) on most measures.

Investigations of neural function, as opposed to structure, in early infancy suggest some abnormalities: there is evidence of either delayed or aberrant auditory system development (Jiang et al. 1990) which might contribute to the widespread hearing disorders observed in DS. Obviously, such a disorder, if organic, could be related to many of the subsequent difficulties seen in the learning of language. Hill Karrer et al. (1998) have reported delayed development of cerebral inhibition using visual event-related potentials (ERP) in a visual recognition memory paradigm. There is also evidence of a more widespread abnormality in EEG coherence (McAlaster 1992) that seems to reflect the generally impoverished dendritic environment (cf. Marin-Padilla 1976). This difference, like many of the others, emerges only some time after birth. It appears that this effect is predominant in posterior, rather than anterior, brain regions, and in the left, more than the right, hemisphere.

The evidence of neuropathological sequellae in DS is more extensive for the middle stage of life. Data from post mortem studies and from studies of brain function in select populations indicate that the changes beginning to emerge early in life become more prominent and prevalent by early adolescence.

There have been relatively few studies of brain function in adolescents and young adults with DS and the existing data are somewhat equivocal. Devinsky et al. (1990) reported relatively normal EEG alpha activity in young adults (<40 years of age), while Schapiro et al. (1992) reported relatively normal brain metabolism in a similar group, using positron emission tomography (PET) measures of glucose uptake and regional blood flow. They did report some disruption of normal neuronal interactions between the frontal and parietal lobes, possibly including the language area of Broca. Overall, they concluded that in younger subjects with DS cerebral atrophy does not generally extend beyond what would be predicted by the smaller cranial vault and stature of these subjects. On the other hand, in those cases where dementia can be observed in younger subjects there are clear signs of abnormal cerebral atrophy and metabolic deficiencies. Enlargement of the ventricles is a standard sign in these cases. In an earlier study looking at glucose uptake these investigators found abnormal interactions between the thalamus and neocortex, in particular the temporal and occipital lobes, speculating that there might be a problem with 'directed attention' as a result (Horwitz et al. 1990).

A PET study of seven young adults with DS (mean age 28 years) without dementia (Haier et al. 1995) confirmed previous findings that overall cortical glucose metabolic rate is higher in subjects with DS (and in other mentally retarded subjects) than in normal controls. This seemingly paradoxical increase is typically interpreted as a sign of 'inefficiency'. When one looks at specific areas more closely, there are decreases in metabolic rate in medial frontal and medial temporal lobes in the DS subjects, and some evidence of dysfunction in the basal ganglia.

Two recent studies (Pinter et al. 2001a; Kates et al. 2002) provide more specific information. Pinter et al. used high-resolution MRI methods to analyse brain structure in 16 youngsters (mean age 11.3 years) with DS. After correcting for overall brain volume, hippocampal but not amygdala volume reductions were seen in this group. This result confirms some earlier work using lower resolution MRI methods (Jernigan et al. 1993). Kates et al. looked at a group of 12 children with DS (all males, mean age 5.94 years) and compared them to children with fragile-X, developmental language delay, or typical development. The children with DS had smaller brain volumes than any of the others, with previously unreported reductions in parietal cortex as well as the oft-reported reductions in the temporal lobe. Pinter et al. (2001b), on the other hand, note the relative preservation of parietal cortex.

Overall, the evidence from the study of subjects in mid-life remains inconclusive. This, however, is not the case when one looks at studies focused on somewhat older subjects. For some time it has been clear that neuropathology resembling that seen in Alzheimer's disease (AD) is prevalent in individuals with DS (DS) after the age of about 35 years. Recent work has explored the ways in which the neuropathology seen in DS is similar to, or different from, that seen in Alzheimer's disease. A very important fact emerging from the past 10 years of careful study is that while virtually 100% of individuals with DS show neuropathology similar to that associated with Alzheimer's disease, less than 50% show the dementia invariably seen with AD (see, for example, Holland et al. 1998). This uncoupling of the neuropathology from the dementia has of course occasioned considerable interest, with an initial emphasis on attempts to determine if there might be subtle differences between the cases of DS and AD that could explain the dissociation observed in DS but not in AD. It has not proven possible to point to any difference that could be said, with confidence, to account for this fact (see, for example, Cork 1990).

Five studies carried out in the 1990s provided data on the neuropathology observed in adults with DS (Weis 1991; Lögdberg & Brun 1993; Kesslak et al. 1994; Raz et al. 1995; Aylward et al. 1999). Weis (1991) demonstrated specific differences in cortex and white matter overall, with a not-quite-significant difference in cerebellum (p < 0.06). The second study (Kesslak et al. 1994) looked at 13 adults with DS, demonstrating a decrease in the size of the hippocampus and neocortex and a paradoxical increase in the size of the parahippocampal gyrus in the group without dementia. No significant differences were observed in the superior temporal lobe, the middle and inferior temporal lobes, the lateral ventricles, or cortical or subcortical areas. In these DS subjects there were only two significant age-related changes: with ageing, ventricle size increased and hippocampal size decreased. In the two subjects with dementia there was considerable brain atrophy and an enlargement of the ventricles; in general there was a picture similar to that observed in Alzheimer's disease, but this was absent in the subjects with DS who were not clinically demented, even those as old as 51 years.

The third study (Raz et al. 1995) looked at 25 adults, 13 with DS, also using MRI. Most critically, their results were adjusted for body size, so they took into account differences resulting simply from allometry. Brain regions that were smaller in the DS subjects included the hippocampal formation, the mammillary bodies, and parts of the cerebellum and cerebral hemispheres. They also replicated the increase in size of the parahippocampal gyrus observed by Kesslak et al. (1994). No differences at all were observed in orbito-frontal cortex, pre- and post-central gyri, and the basal ganglia. The fourth study (Lögdberg & Brun 1993) applied morphometric analyses to the brains of seven subjects with DS (mean age of 25.3 years) and demonstrated a significant decrease in gyri in the frontal lobe. Finally, Aylward et al. (1999) used high-resolution MRI to show a selective hippocampal volume reduction in adults.

These observed changes confirm earlier reports of decreased volume of cerebellum (Jernigan & Bellugi 1990), and of decreased dendritic spines and volume in hippocampus (Ferrer & Gullotta 1990). There have also been reports of neuropathology in the amygdala (Mann & Esiri 1989; Murphy et al. 1992), in particular in those subregions most closely associated with the hippocampus (Murphy & Ellis 1991) but the more recent findings that controlled for overall brain volume (Pinter et al. 2001a) cast some doubt on these data.

The earliest neuropathological changes with ageing in DS seem to appear in parts of the hippocampal formation, especially the entorhinal cortex, but also involving the dentate gyrus, CA1 and the subiculum (Mann & Esiri 1989; Hyman 1992). There is extensive cell loss in the locus coeruleus (Mann et al. 1990), a brainstem nucleus that projects to the hippocampal formation; this was most noticeable in cases of severe dementia.

In sum, there are widespread signs of neuropathology in older subjects with DS but there is selectivity, nonetheless, in terms of where signs are seen first, and where they are most prominent. In this regard, changes in hippocampal formation (Ball & Nuttal 1981; Sylvester 1983; Ball et al. 1986), temporal lobe in general (Deb et al. 1992; Spargo et al. 1992), prefrontal cortex (Logdberg & Brun 1993; Kesslak et al. 1994) and cerebellum (Cole et al. 1993) stand out.

Overall, study of neuropathology in early and later life points to certain regions of the cortex, including most prominently the temporal lobe and the hippocampal formation (Wisniewski et al. 1986), the prefrontal cortex, and the cerebellum. In analysing learning and memory difficulties we should be particularly alert to changes that reflect problems with these neural systems. There is a substantial and growing literature dealing with the hippocampal system and prefrontal cortex in DS but the possible role of the cerebellum has generally been downplayed. Given the persistent abnormalities observed in this structure closer examination of its role in the behavioural and cognitive phenotype in DS should be a high priority for the future.

DOWN SYNDROME COMPARED TO OTHER MR SYNDROMES

It is worth noting that the pattern of neuropathology observed in DS is quite specific to this case – other MR syndromes present a rather different picture. In Williams syndrome, for example, there is relative sparing of the frontal and limbic regions affected in DS, with deficits in cortical areas underlying language and face perception (Bellugi et al. 1999). In fragile-X, increases in hippocampal, thalamic and caudate volume have been observed along with preservation of parietal white matter (Kates et al. 2002). In yet another syndrome, autism, a still different picture emerges with defects observed more widely in hippocampus, subiculum, entorhinal cortex, septal nuclei, mamillary body, selected nuclei of the amygdala, neocerebellar cortex, roof nuclei of the cerebellum, and inferior olivary nucleus (Bauman & Kemper 1985). These important differences in the neuropathology observed across various MR syndromes strongly suggest that the cognitive defects observed in these syndromes should also differ, with each syndrome demonstrating a specific pattern of spared and impaired function.

COGNITION IN INDIVIDUALS WITH DS

In general, infants with DS show relatively normal abilities in learning and memory (but see Hepper & Shahidullah 1992 for a report of impaired habituation in two foetuses with DS). It is essential to understand, however, that this does not mean that either they, or indeed normally developing infants, have the full adult range of learning and memory abilities at birth. In fact this is not the case because some parts of the brain mature postnatally and the forms of learning and memory dependent on them are not available until some time after birth. The medial temporal lobe, and particularly the hippocampus, as well as parts of the cerebellum, are included in this category. The fact that these late-developing structures are apparently particularly at risk in DS is probably of considerable importance (see Nadel 1986).

In an early series of studies, Ohr & Fagen (1991, 1993) reported that 3-month-old infants with DS were entirely normal in learning about the contingencies between their own movements (leg kicking) and reinforcement, including initial learning, acquisition speed and retention. In a later report, Ohr & Fagen (1994) showed that 9-month-old infants with DS were impaired, as a group, in learning about the contingency between arm movements and reinforcement. However, they noted that some infants with DS were able to learn. They concluded that there is a relative decline in conditionability in infants with DS compared to normally developing infants after 6 months.

Mangan (1992) tested control infants and infants with DS on a variety of spatial tasks, one of which, a place-learning task, was designed especially to assess the state of function of the hippocampal system. The pattern of results was consistent with diffuse, but mild, neuropathology combined with much more extensive pathology localised to the hippocampus.

A great deal of work on learning within the language domain has been carried out in children with DS (see Rondal 1994). There is little doubt that difficulties in the acquisition of language can be quite severe, particularly in the phonological and syntactic domains (see Tager-Flusberg 1999; Vicari et al. 2002; Thordardottir et al. 2002), but there are also cases where language capacity is within normal range, or even at the upper end of that range. Infants with DS show many of the normal features of prelanguage behaviour, including babbling and imitation, although there are some subtle but possibly important differences between DS and normally developing infants in this regard (Oller & Siebert 1988; Lynch et al. 1990; Steffens et al. 1992).

Sigman and her colleagues (Mundy et al. 1988; Sigman 1999) have shown deficits in the use of nonverbal requests in young children with DS.

Similar deficits in requesting behaviour have been seen in other studies, including one assessing verbal requests (Beeghly et al. 1990), but a number of studies have failed to detect a deficit (for example, Greenwald & Leonard 1979). Vocalisation appears to be under contingent control in infants with DS (Poulson 1988), and their ability to acquire words seems normal as well, although slow (Hopmann & Nothnagle 1994). While it is hard to pinpoint the precise defect at the root of the typical language problem, there is little to suggest that the difficulty is primarily one of learning or memory. Sigman (1999) stresses defective requesting behaviour, less-than-optimal caregiver behaviour, and diminished capacity to initiate joint attention as precursors to language problems. Tager-Flusberg (1999) focuses on auditory working memory, which certainly could account for the observed phonological defects. The fact that disproportionate difficulties are observed in grammatical development is consistent with the idea that learning and memory problems are not at the root of language defects in DS.

Young children develop notions about the continuing existence and properties of objects in a characteristic fashion. Children with DS have typically been shown to acquire this basic object concept more slowly than normal (see, for example, Rast & Meltzoff 1995) but with extensive training they can acquire it at more-or-less the same time as normally developing infants (Wishart 1993). However, a different kind of problem emerges in this task situation: instability of acquisition. Although the typical subject with DS solved various levels of the tasks used to assess the object concept at ages not very far from the norm, performance after acquisition could be highly variable and apparently beset by motivational difficulties. These problems, if representative of the learning style of children with DS, are extremely important in thinking about effective intervention. The results of Wishart's studies using standard intelligence test batteries suggest that they are indeed representative. Test-retest reliability was very low because successes gained in one test might not appear upon retest, as soon as 2 weeks later. New skills show up, only to disappear shortly thereafter. One could speculate that evidence of such 'rapid forgetting' is consistent with damage in the hippocampal formation but considerably more data are required before this conclusion can be accepted.

The motivational difficulties and developmental instabilities observed in Wishart's work strongly suggest that young children with DS are not merely delayed in mental development, but actually follow a somewhat different path. As Wishart (1993, p. 392) points out, this view 'has the substantial merit of being consistent with data from the neurosciences showing DS to be associated with fundamental differences in the morphology and functioning of the brain.'

To summarise the situation in infants and children: there is evidence of relatively normal learning of certain types, especially in the youngest subjects.

The kinds of learning that appear normal fall into the category often referred to as 'procedural': simple conditioning, for example, and deferred imitation (Rast & Meltzoff 1995). There is also evidence for some highly specific learning deficits, which typically emerge only some months or even years after birth. The evidence is consistent with a specific problem in the hippocampal formation spatial cognitive system.

The learning and memory problems that begin to emerge in late infancy become considerably more noticeable as the infant grows to childhood and adolescence. While much of our knowledge for this period comes from the learning of language, there is information available about other kinds of learning and memory. One major point to be stressed from these language learning data has less to do with the inability of children with DS to acquire words, or linguistic constructions, or other non-verbal material, and more to do with their inability to 'stabilise' the information that they do manage to acquire. Wishart (1993) and Fowler (1988) stress this point, which might reflect, among other factors, impairments in memory consolidation, another function of the hippocampal system.

In one of the earliest studies taking into account the multiple forms of learning and memory, Carlesimo et al. (1997) reported a selective impairment in DS. Subjects with DS were tested on a variety of 'implicit' (procedural) and 'explicit' (episodic) memory paradigms, including word-stem completion, list learning and prose recall. Robust priming effects were seen in the DS group, comparable to those observed in controls, indicating that implicit memory was intact. However, deficits were observed in both explicit memory tasks. Performance on these kinds of explicit memory paradigms has been linked to functions of the hippocampal system, hence the defects suggest differential impairment in hippocampal function and thereby converge with the data from study of spatial cognition.

In a series of recent studies my colleagues and I have tested several different groups of individuals with DS on a range of tasks designed to directly assess the function of specific brain systems. This 'cognitive neuropsychological' approach often uses tasks first developed in animal models, where the critical underlying brain circuits can be identified and carefully studied in invasive experiments. We started with a focus on three brain systems identified by the neuropathological data, much of which was discussed above: the hippocampal system, the prefrontal cortex, and the cerebellum. We developed a set of tasks that could, collectively, tell us something about how these brain systems are faring. In the first set of studies (Pennington et al. 2003) we found evidence of specific hippocampal dysfunction in our sample of 28 adolescents, using mental age matched controls. We found little evidence of prefrontal dysfunction in a battery of nonverbal tasks. Subsequent pilot work, however, suggested that verbal tasks might yield a different result, and indeed that is what we are now seeing (Moon et al., in preparation). Using verbal tasks to explore the prefrontal cortex, we found in our young and old groups strong signs of dysfunction in both the hippocampal and prefrontal systems. Deficits were observed in a range of tasks although verbal mediation was necessary to bring out the prefrontal effect. Taken as a whole, our studies show that particular problems emerge in the memory domains served by the hippocampal system and the prefrontal system. The latter impairment appears to be linked to the use of verbal test materials. The impairment in hippocampal function could in principle reflect problems in any of the structures of the hippocampal region; a recent study of two neuropsychological paradigms dependent on parahippocampal and perirhinal regions (delayed nonmatching to sample and visual paired comparison), however, suggests that these areas are functioning appropriately, and that the impairment is more likely to reflect improper development of the hippocampus itself (Dawson et al. 2001).

The prefrontal cortex, as noted already, plays an important role in a wide range of functions, including episodic/explicit memory and working memory. We have already seen that episodic memory is impaired in individuals with DS. There has been extensive research on working memory in this population, and clear deficits have been observed in a number of studies (Varnhagen et al. 1987; Marcell & Weeks 1988; Laws 1998; Jarrold et al. 2000, 2002). However, this impairment seems to be limited to verbal information, as impairments are minimal in visuospatial domains. The deficit appears to be neither a motor nor articulatory problem (Kanno & Ikeda 2002) and may relate to the so-called phonological loop (Laws 2002).

Thus, several forms of data indicate that specific impairments in prefrontal cortex and the hippocampal system are an important part of the phenotype of DS. This suggests a framework for research in the future: what is it about an extra chromosome 21 that leads to particular impairments in the function of these two particular systems?

COGNITIVE FUNCTION IN DS COMPARED TO OTHER MR SYNDROMES

As noted earlier, the pattern of neural impairments differs across MR syndromes. Thus, it is not surprising that the pattern of cognitive impairments should do so as well. Table 5.1 displays the pattern observed in DS – which functions are relatively spared and which relatively impaired.

Table 5.1 shows that the pattern of impairments and sparing is highly selective – some aspects of memory are relatively normal, others are quite impaired. Some forms of spatial cognition are normal, others impaired.

If one compares this picture to what is observed in other forms of MR, one sees again that the patterns are quite different. For example, children with WS do not show specific difficulties with morphosyntactic aspects of language (Vicari et al. 2002). They are, however, impaired in verbal learning tasks (Nichols et al. 2004) and show delayed, atypical development in all areas of

Table 5.1. Cognitive functions relatively spared and impaired in Down syndrome

Relatively spared	Relatively impaired
Visual short-term memory	Auditory short-term memory
Implicit memory	Phonology
Conditioning	Morpho-syntax
Social cognition	Explicit memory
Theory of mind	Memory consolidation
Deferred imitation	Allocentric space
Object concept	Finger coordination
Egocentric space	

language function (Donnai & Karmiloff-Smith 2000). Auditory short-term memory is impaired in DS, but relatively preserved in WS. In the perceptual domain, children with WS are particularly impaired on global organisation, whereas children with DS have difficulties with local organisation. Even when performance is impaired in both groups, as in block-design tasks, the nature of the impairment differs (see Bellugi et al. 1999 for a review).

Differentiations also emerge when DS is compared to another MR syndrome – Prader-Willi. In contrast with children with DS, who are generally quite good in terms of social skills, children with Prader-Willi syndrome exhibit a pattern of social impairments, including extreme sensitivity, anxiety, and obsessive-compulsive behaviours (Walz & Benson 2002).

Thus, each MR syndrome seems to be characterised by a specific set of cognitive impairments, presumably reflecting the unique neural defects underlying that syndrome. One obvious implication of this fact is that intervention strategies will have to be tailored specifically for each syndrome.

CONCLUSIONS

Cognition is disrupted in DS and progress is being made in defining exactly what the deficit is. Most indications suggest that the impairment is not spread across all systems equally but instead selectively impacts only some systems. This pattern of selective impairment differs between MR syndromes. What is observed in DS is quite unlike what is observed in other syndromes, such as WS, fragile-X, or Prader-Willi syndrome.

There is at this time clear evidence for DS implicating forms of cognition dependent upon the hippocampus; strong evidence implicating the prefrontal cortex is also available. No doubt other impairments will be found, most probably including the cerebellum, or parts of the cerebellum. This research has provided a reasonably clear picture of which aspects of improper neural development might be responsible for the particular features of the mental retardation seen in DS.

How do we go from this kind of knowledge to an understanding of the linkage between the genetic defect and the neural and cognitive phenotype emerging in these studies of DS? Our current strategy is to identify as carefully as possible the neural and cognitive phenotype in humans with DS, differentiating it carefully from the mental retardation observed in other syndromes. Then, one can try to create mouse models that isolate just those genes responsible for the specific features of the DS phenotype. By paying careful attention to what is unique about DS we enhance our ability to uncover its source, and hence our ability to do something to ameliorate the most severe consequences of this form of mental retardation.

REFERENCES

Aylward, E. H., Li, Q., Honeycutt, N. A., Warren, A. C., Pulsifer, M. B., Barta, P. E., et al. (1999) MRI volumes of the hippocampus and amygdala in adults with Down's syndrome with and without dementia. *Am J Psychiatr*, **156**, 564–568.

Ball, M. J., Nuttall, K. (1981) Topography of neurofibrillary tangles and granovacuoles in the hippocampi of patients with Down's syndrome: Quantitative comparison with normal ageing and Alzheimer's disease. *Neuropathol Appl Neurobiol*, **7**, 13–20.

Ball, M. J., Schapiro, M. B., Rapoport, S. I. (1986) Neuropathological relationships between Down syndrome and senile dementia Alzheimer type. In C. J. Epstein (ed.) *The Neurobiology of Down Syndrome*. New York: Raven Press, pp. 45–58.

Bar-Peled, O., Israeli, M., Ben-Hur, H., Hoskins, I., Groner, Y., Biegon, A. (1991) Developmental patterns of muscarinic receptors in normal and Down's syndrome fetal brain – an autoradiographic study. *Neurosci Lett*, **133**, 154–158.

Bauman, M., Kemper, T. L. (1985) Histoanatomic observations of the brain in early infantile autism. *Neurology*, **35**, 866–874.

Becker, L. E., Armstrong, D. L., Chan, F. (1986) Dendritic atrophy in children with Down's syndrome. *Ann Neurol*, **20**, 520–526.

Beeghly, M., Weiss-Perry, B., Cicchetti, D. (1990) Beyond sensorimotor functioning: early communicative and play development of children with Down syndrome. In D. Cicchetti, M. Beeghly (eds) *Children with Down Syndrome: A Developmental Perspective*. New York: Cambridge University Press, pp. 329–368.

Bellugi, U., Lichtenberger, L., Mills, D., Galaburda, A., Korenberg, J. R. (1999) Bridging cognition, the brain and molecular genetics: evidence from Williams syndrome. *Trends in Neuroscience*, **22**, 197–207.

Benda, C. E. (1971) Mongolism. In J. Minckler (ed.) *Pathology of the Nervous System*, Vol. 2. New York: McGraw-Hill, p. 1867.

Blackwood, W., Corsellis, J. A. N. (1976) *Greenfield's Neuropathology*. Chicago: Yearbook Medical, pp. 420–421.

Brooksbank, B. W. L., Walker, D., Balazs, R., Jorgensen, O. S. (1989) Neuronal maturation in the foetal brain in Down syndrome. *Early Hum Dev*, **18**, 237–246.

Carlesimo, G. A., Marotta, L., Vicari, S. (1997) Long-term memory in mental retardation: evidence for a specific impairment in subjects with Down's syndrome. *Neuropsychologia*, **35**, 71–79.

Cole, G., Neal, J. W., Singhrao, S. K., Jasani, B., Newman, G. R. (1993) The distribution of amyloid plaques in the cerebellum and brain stem in Down's syndrome and Alzheimer's disease: a light microscopical analysis. *Acta Neuropathol*, **85**, 542–552.

Cork, L. C. (1990) Neuropathology of Down syndrome and Alzheimer disease. *Am J Med Genet Suppl*, **7**, 282–286.

Crome, L., Cowie, V., Slater, E. (1966) A statistical note on cerebellar and brain-stem weight in Mongolism. *J Ment Defic*, **10**, 69–72.

Dawson, G., Osterling, J., Rinaldi, J., Carver, L., McPartland, J. (2001) Brief Report: recognition memory and stimulus-reward associations: indirect support for the role of ventromedial prefrontal dysfunction in autism. *J Autism Dev Disord*, **31**, 337–341.

Deb, S., De Silva, P. N., Gemmell, H. G., Besson, J. A. O., Smith, F. W., Ebmeier, K. P. (1992) Alzheimer's disease in adults with Down's syndrome: the relationship between regional cerebral blood flow equivalents and dementia. *Acta Psychiatr Scand*, **86**, 340–345.

Devinsky, O., Sato, S., Conwit, R. A., Schapiro, M. B. (1990) Relation of EEG alpha background to cognitive function, brain atrophy, and cerebral metabolism in Down's syndrome. *Arch Neurol*, **47**, 58–62.

Donnai, D., Karmiloff-Smith, A. (2000) Williams syndrome: from genotype through to the cognitive phenotype. *Am J Med Genet: Seminars in Medical Genetics*, **97**, 164–171.

Engidawork, E., Lubec, G. (2003) Molecular changes in fetal Down syndrome brain. *J Neurochem*, **84**, 895–904.

Ferrer, I., Gullotta, F. (1990) Down's syndrome and Alzheimer's disease: dendritic spine counts in hippocampus. *Acta Neuropathol*, **79**, 680–685.

Flórez, J., Del Arco, C., Gonzalez, A., Pascual, J., Pazos, A. (1990) Autoradiographic studies of neurotransmitter receptors in the brain of newborn infants with Down syndrome. *Am J Med Genet Suppl*, **7**, 301–305.

Fowler, A. (1988) Determinants of rate of language growth in children with DS. In L. Nadel (ed.) *The Psychobiology of Down Syndrome*. Cambridge MA: MIT Press, pp. 215–245.

Golden, J. A., Hyman, B. T. (1994) Development of the superior temporal neocortex is anomalous in trisomy 21. *J Neuropathol Exp Neurol*, **53**, 513–520.

Greenwald, C. A., Leonard, L. (1979) Communicative and sensorimotor development of Down's syndrome children. *Am J Ment Defic*, **84**, 296–303.

Haier, R. J., Chueh, D., Touchette, P., Lott, I., Buchsbaum, M.S., MacMillan, D., et al. (1995) Brain size and cerebral glucose metabolic rate in non-specific mental retardation and Down syndrome. *Intelligence*, **20**, 191–210.

Hepper, P. G., Shahidullah, S. (1992) Habituation in Normal and Down's syndrome fetuses. *Q J Exp Psychol*, **44B**, 305–317.

Hill Karrer, J., Karrer, R., Bloom, D., Chaney, L., Davis, R. (1998) Event-related brain potentials during an extended visual recognition memory task depict delayed development of cerebral inhibitory processes among 6-month-old infants with Down syndrome. *Int J Psychophysiol*, **29**, 167–200.

Holland, A. J., Hon, J., Huppert, F., Stevens, F., Watson, P. (1998) Population-based study of the prevalence and presentation of dementia in adults with Down's syndrome. *Br J Psychiatr*, **172**, 493–498.

Hopmann, M. R., Nothnagle, M. B. (1994) A longitudinal study of early vocabulary of infants with Down syndrome and infants who are developing normally. Poster presented at International Down syndrome Research Conference, Charleston, South Carolina, April 1994.

Horwitz, B., Schapiro, M. B., Grady, C. L., Rapoport, S. I. (1990) Cerebral metabolic pattern in young adult Down's syndrome subjects: altered intercorrelations between regional rates of glucose utilization. *J Ment Defic Res*, **34**, 237–252.

Hyman, B. T. (1992) Down syndrome and Alzheimer disease. In L. Nadel and C. J. Epstein (eds) *Down Syndrome and Alzheimer Disease*. New York: Wiley-Liss, pp. 123–142.

Jarrold, C., Baddeley, A. D., Hewes, A. K. (2000) Verbal short-term memory deficits in Down syndrome, a consequence of problems in rehearsal? *J Child Psychol Psychiatr*, **41**, 233–244.

Jernigan, T. L., Bellugi, U. (1990) Anomalous brain morphology on magnetic resonance images in Williams syndrome and Down syndrome. *Arch Neurol*, **47**, 529–533.

Jernigan, T. L., Bellugi, U., Sowell, E., Doherty, S., Hesselink, J. R. (1993) Cerebral morphological distinctions between Williams and Down syndrome. *Arch Neurol*, **50**, 186–191.

Jiang, Z. D., Wu, Y. Y., Liu, X. Y. (1990) Early development of brainstem auditory evoked potentials in Down's syndrome. *Early Hum Dev*, **23**, 41–51.

Kanno, K., Ikeda, Y. (2002) Word-length effect in verbal short-term memory in individuals with Down's syndrome. *J Intellect Disabil Res*, **46**, 613–618.

Kates, W. R., Folley, B. S., Lanham, D. C., Capone, G. T., Kaufmann, W. E. (2002) Cerebral growth in Fragile X syndrome: review and comparison with Down syndrome. *Microsc Res Tech*, **57**, 159–167.

Kesslak, J. P., Nagata, S. F., Lott, I., Nalcioglu, O. (1994) Magnetic resonance imaging analysis of age-related changes in the brains of individuals with Down's syndrome. *Neurology*, **44**, 1039–1045.

Koo, B., Blaser, S., Harwood-Nash, D., Becker, L., Murphy, E. G. (1992) Magnetic resonance imaging evaluation of delayed myelination in Down syndrome: a case report and review of the literature. *J Child Neurol*, **7**, 417–421.

Laws, G. (1998) The use of nonword repetition as a test of phonological memory in children with Down syndrome. *J Child Psychol Psychiatr*, **39**, 1119–1130.

Laws, G. (2002) Working memory in children and adolescents with Down syndrome: evidence from a colour memory experiment. *J Child Psychol Psychiatr*, **43**, 353–364.

Lögdberg, B., Brun, A. (1993) Prefrontal neocortical disturbances in mental retardation. *J Intellect Disabil Res*, **37**, 459–468.

Lynch, M., Oller, K., Eilers, R., Basinger, D. (1990) Vocal development of infants with Down's syndrome. Symposium for Research on Child Language Disorders, Madison, WI.

Mangan, P. A. (1992) Spatial memory abilities and abnormal development of the hippocampal formation in Down syndrome. Unpublished doctoral dissertation, University of Arizona, Tucson.

Mann, D. M. A., Esiri, M. M. (1989) The pattern of acquisition of plaques and tangles in the brains of patients under 50 years of age with Down's syndrome. *J Neurol Sci*, **89**, 169–179.

Mann, D. M. A., Royston, M. C., Ravindra, C. R. (1990) Some morphometric observations on the brains of patients with Down's syndrome: their relationship to age and dementia. *J Neurol Sci*, **99**, 153–164.

Marcell, M. M. Weeks, S. L. (1988) Short-term memory difficulties and Down's syndrome. *J Ment Def Res*, **32**, 153–162.

Marin-Padilla, M. (1976) Pyramidal cell abnormalities in the motor cortex of a child with Down's syndrome. A Golgi study. *J Comp Nerurol*, **167**, 63–81.

McAlaster, R. (1992) Postnatal cerebral maturation in Down's syndrome children: a developmental EEG coherence study. *Int J Neurosci*, **65**, 221–237.

Mundy, P., Sigman, M., Kasari, C., Yirmiya, N. (1988) Nonverbal communication skills in Down syndrome children. *Child Dev*, **59**, 235–249.

Murphy, G. M. Jr. and Ellis, W. G. (1991) The amygdala in Down's syndrome and familial Alzheimer's disease: four clinicopathological case reports. *Biol Psychiatr*, **30**, 92–106.

Murphy, G. M. Jr., Ellis, W. G., Lee, Y.-L., Stultz, K. E., Shrivastava, R., Tinklenberg, J. R., et al. (1992) Astrocytic gliosis in the amygdala in Down's syndrome and Alzheimer's disease. In A. C. H. Yu, L. Hertz, M. D. Norenberg, E. Sykova, S.G. Waxman (eds) *Progress in Brain Research*, Vol. 94. Amsterdam: Elsevier Science Publishers, pp. 475–483.

Nadel, L. (1986) Down syndrome in neurobiological perspective. In C. J. Epstein (ed.) *The Neurobiology of Down Syndrome*. New York: Raven Press, pp. 239–251.

Nichols, S., Jones, W., Roman, M. J., Wulfeck, B., Delis, D. C., Reilly, J., Bellugi, U. (2004) Mechanisms of verbal memory impairment in four neurodevelopmental disorders. *Brain Lang*, **88**, 180–189.

Ohr, P. S., Fagen, J. W. (1991) Conditioning and long-term memory in three-month-old infants with Down syndrome. *Am J Ment Retard*, **96**, 151–162.

Ohr, P. S., Fagen, J. W. (1993) Temperament, conditioning, and memory in 3-month-old infants with Down syndrome. *J Appl Dev Psychol*, **14**, 175–190.

Ohr, P. S., Fagen, J. W. (1994) Contingency learning in 9-month-old infants with Down syndrome. *Am J Ment Retard*, **99**, 74–84.

O'Keefe, J., Nadel, L. (1978) *The Hippocampus as a Cognitive Map*. Oxford: Clarendon Press.

Oller, K., Siebert, J. M. (1988) Babbling in prelinguistic retarded children. *Am J Ment Retard*, **92**, 369–375.

Pazos, A., Del Olmo, E., Diaz, A., Del Arco, C., Rodriguez-Puertas, R., Pascual, J., et al. (1994) Serotonergic (5-HT$_{1A}$ and 5-HT$_{1D}$) and muscarinic cholinergic receptors in DS brains: an autoradiographic analysis. Poster presented at International Down syndrome Research Conference, Charleston, South Carolina, April 1994.

Pennington, B. F., Moon, J., Edgin, J., Stedron, J., Nadel, L. (2003) The neuropsychology of Down syndrome: evidence for hippocampal dysfunction. *Child Dev*, **74**, 75–93.

Pinter, J. D., Brown, W. E., Eliez, S., Schmitt, J. E., Capone, G. T., Reiss, A. L. (2001a) Amygdala and hippocampal volumes in children with Down syndrome: a high-resolution MRI study. *Neurology*, **56**, 972–974.

Pinter, J. D., Eliez, S., Schmitt, E., Capone, G., Reiss, A. L. (2001b) Neuroanatomy of Down's syndrome: a high-resolution MRI study. *Am J Psychiat*, **158**, 1659–1665.

Poulson, C. L. (1988) Operant conditioning of vocalization rate of infants with Down syndrome. *Am J Ment Retard*, **93**, 57–63.

Rast, M., Meltzoff, A. N. (1995) Memory and representation in young children with Down syndrome: exploring deferred imitation and object permanence. *Dev Psychopathol*, **7**, 393–407.

Raz, N., Torres, I. J., Briggs, S. D., Spencer, W. D., Thornton, A. E., Loken, W. J., et al. (1995) Selective neuroanatomical abnormalities in Down syndrome and their cognitive correlates: evidence from MRI morphometry. *Neurology*, **45**, 356–366.

Rondal, J. A. (1994) Exceptional language development in mental retardation: the relative autonomy of language as a cognitive system. In H. Tager-Flusberg (ed.) *Constraints on Language Acquisition: Studies of Atypical Children*. Hillsdale NJ: Erlbaum, pp. 155–174.

Schapiro, M. B., Haxby, J. V., Grady, C. L. (1992) Nature of mental retardation and dementia in Down syndrome: study with PET, CT, and neuropsychology. *Neurobiology of Aging*, **13**, 723–734.

Schmidt-Sidor, B., Wisniewski, K., Shepard, T. H., Sersen, E. A. (1990) Brain growth in Down syndrome subjects 15 to 22 weeks of gestational age and birth to 60 months. *Clin Neuropathol*, **9**, 181–190.

Sigman, M. (1999) Developmental deficits in children with Down syndrome. In H. Tager-Flusberg (ed.) *Neurodevelopmental Disorders*. Cambridge MA: MIT Press, pp. 179–196.

Spargo, E., Luthert, P. J., Janota, I., Lantos, P. L. (1992) ß4A deposition in the temporal cortex of adults with Down's syndrome. *J Neurol Sci*, **111**, 26–32.

Steffens, M. L., Oller, K., Lynch, M., Urbano, R. (1992) Vocal development in infants with Down syndrome and infants who are developing normally. *Am J Ment Retard*, **97**, 235–246.

Sylvester, P. E. (1983) The hippocampus in Down's syndrome. *J Mental Def Res*, **27**, 227–236.

Tager-Flusberg, H. (ed.) (1999) *Neurodevelopmental Disorders*. Cambridge MA: MIT Press.

Thordardottir, E. T., Chapman, R. S., Wagner, L. (2002) Complex sentence production by adolescents with Down syndrome. *Applied Psycholinguistics*, **23**, 163–183.

Varnhagen, C. K., Das, J. P., Varnhagen, S. (1987) Auditory and visual memory span: cognitive processing by TMR individuals with Down syndrome or other etiologies. *Am J Ment Def*, **91**, 398–405.

Vicari, S., Caselli, M. C., Gagliardi, C., Tonucci, F., Volterra, V. (2002) Language acquisition in special populations: a comparison between Down and Williams syndromes. *Neuropsychologia*, **40**, 2461–2470.

Walz, N. C., Benson, B. A. (2002) Behavioral phenotypes in children with Down syndrome, Prader-Willi syndrome, or Angelman syndrome. *J Dev Phys Disabil*, **14**, 307–321.

Weis, S. (1991) Morphometry and magnetic resonance imaging of the human brain in normal controls and Down's syndrome. *Anat Rec*, **231**, 593–598.

Wishart, J. (1993) The development of learning difficulties in children with Down syndrome. *J Intellect Disabil Res*, **37**, 389–403.

Wisniewski, K. (1990) Down syndrome children often have brain with maturation delay, retardation of growth, and cortical dysgenesis. *Am J Med Genet Suppl*, **7**, 274–281.

Wisniewski, K., Kida, E. (1994) Abnormal neurogenesis and synaptogenesis in Down syndrome. *Development and Brain Dysfunction*, **7**, 289–301.

Wisniewski, K., Laure-Kamionowska, M., Connell, F., Wen, G. Y. (1986) Neuronal density and synaptogenesis in the postnatal stage of brain maturation in Down syndrome. In C. J. Epstein (ed.) *The Neurobiology of Down Syndrome*. New York: Raven Press, pp. 29–44.

Wisniewski, K., Schmidt-Sidor, B. (1989) Postnatal delay of myelin formation in brains from Down syndrome infants and children. *Clin Neuropathol*, **8**, 55–62.

6 The Contribution of Memory to the Behavioural Phenotype of Down Syndrome

DARLYNNE A. DEVENNY

Institute for Basic Research in Developmental Disabilities, New York, USA

SUMMARY

Memory in adolescents and young adults with Down syndrome (DS) shows a characteristic profile. Implicit memory (memory for procedures and for experiences that do not require deliberate or effortful cognitive processes) and semantic memory (memory for the meanings of words and for knowledge) appear to be commensurate with their overall level of functioning. Working memory (temporary maintenance and manipulation of information) appears to be more severely impaired for auditory-verbal material than for visuospatial material. Episodic memory (memory for events located in a specific time and place) spans a longer duration than working memory and is impaired in both the verbal and spatial domains.

These specific strengths and weaknesses in memory are characteristic of a DS phenotype, although the biological basis for the profile is not clear at this time. In general, memory ability is related to developmental and experiential changes in the nervous system and is sensitive to the rate and characteristics of development in other domains (such as language and cognition). The profile of memory associated with DS, then, will be modified across the lifespan, depending on the interaction of many developmental processes and life experiences, some of which are unique to this syndrome. In addition to systematic developmental changes, within any group of individuals with DS there is considerable variability in performance on memory and other cognitive tasks, making it difficult to predict performance capabilities and the trajectory of development of any specific individual. Understanding the sources of this variability will be critical in revealing relationships between memory processes and cognition in individuals with DS.

Down Syndrome: Neurobehavioural Specificity. Edited by JA Rondal and J Perera.
© 2006 John Wiley & Sons Ltd.

Memory is responsive to life experiences, so within this system there is the possibility for modification through intervention. It is important that research first address issues related to the fundamental processes of memory in individuals with DS and their interactions with other components of cognition and then develop programmes of remediation to facilitate compensation for areas of deficit.

INTRODUCTION

What is memory for? In a most general sense, memory is the imperfect but unique history of an individual. The imprints of our past experiences are contained in memory, including what we have done, the people and places we have known, the ideas that have captured our attention, things we have learned, feelings we have had. These recorded experiences are formative, both from the perspective of personal history and as signposts that guide our future actions and thoughts. Memory also has a role in active thinking. Ideas or items are brought into awareness from stored information and are actively processed and manipulated to produce plans of action, new perspectives or ideas.

Contemporary neuropsychology has demonstrated the utility of employing a systems approach to the study of memory (Squire 1987; Schacter & Tulving 1994), even though it is recognised that the boundaries between the memory system components are not always clearly demarcated. Recognising that the memory processes of individuals with mental retardation (MR) may be influenced by many factors in somewhat unique ways related to the aetiology of their developmental disability, the taxonomy of memory systems is nevertheless broadly applicable to individuals with and without MR. Within the taxonomy of memory systems, one distinction is between *explicit* memory, which is memory that is intentional and effortful, and *implicit* memory, which is memory that is relatively unintentional and automatic. (Other terms include declarative and non-declarative memory, respectively.)

Several components have been described within the division of explicit memory, each corresponding to relatively discrete processes that have both structural and functional properties. The first component, *working memory*, is the description given to the processes that extract information from the environment or from personal knowledge and maintain it in consciousness temporarily so it can be manipulated during comprehension, learning and reasoning. Working memory is related to the conscious awareness of immediate events taking place. Holding a thought, a location, or a fact in awareness while attending to and integrating subsequent incoming information is necessary for coherent action in everyday situations.

In the model of working memory originally proposed by Baddeley and his associates (1986) there were three components. Temporary storage with limited capacity is represented by two slave systems: (1) the *auditory/phono-logical loop* has priority access to the processing of phonological information and briefly retains this verbal information in a buffer until it is used; (2) the *visuospatial sketchpad* is a comparable component that briefly retains visual and spatial information. A third component of the model, (3) the *central executive*, exercises control over processing of information and controls attention to the incoming information. Recently a fourth component, (4) an *episodic buffer*, which is capable of integrating information from many sources, including information from memory in long-term storage that is pertinent to the task at hand, was added to the model (Baddeley 2000, 2001).

The second component of explicit memory, *episodic memory*, is the registering of information that is identified with a specific time and place (Tulving 1983) although it is dependent on the knowledge base of previously learned meanings and situations. Episodic memory spans a time frame of minutes to years, as compared to working memory, which has a time frame of seconds unless strategies are employed (such as rehearsal) to prolong the memory trace. Long-term consolidation of this type of memory depends on the integrity of the hippocampus and its reciprocal connections to the frontal lobes. The broader functions of episodic memory are directly related to autobiographical memory. Our sense of self is formed, in large part, from the accumulation of our unique remembered experiences and their effects on our emotional and cognitive functioning.

Semantic memory, yet another component of explicit memory, is associated with the organisation of our general knowledge of the world and includes word meanings, concepts and symbols (Tulving 1983). This memory component is characterised by very long-term retention and an almost unlimited capacity. While episodic memory is related to personal experience, semantic memory is related to the transmission of cultural and accumulated knowledge.

Finally, there is the type of memory in which knowledge and skills are gained through routines, practice and prior exposure, the type of memory that we are able to use without conscious effort. *Implicit memory* refers to the influence or facilitation of a specific experience on memory without the support of deliberate or effortful retrieval processes (Graf & Schacter 1985; Schacter 1987). Implicit memory supports much of our daily routinised functioning such as the memory for the movements involved in riding a bicycle. Implicit memory also has several subcomponents including classical and operant conditioning, procedural knowledge (the sequence of moves necessary to reproduce a rule-governed pattern) and priming (facilitation based on prior exposure).

Thus memory is clearly not a single entity. It represents the integration of all the described subcomponents within a dynamic system and is interdependent with other components of cognition (such as attention and reasoning) and language. Indeed, much of memory is encoded through language. The tenses of language mark elements of time that presuppose a memory of the past and how it is distinguished from the present. Memory allows us to think about the future and adapt to future expectations because we have an awareness of having experienced a past (Tulving 2002).

Anecdotal observations of individuals with DS have suggested that there are discrepancies in their ability within the domain of memory. Oster (1953, reported in Gibson 1978) commented on their ability to remember persons and situations while having difficulty retaining a brief message. Despite historical observations such as this, the syndrome-specific study of memory has been relatively recent. Although many earlier studies of individuals with MR undoubtedly included individuals with DS, their performance within the subject group was not distinguished (for example, Belmont 1966; Ellis 1970; Ellis et al. 1970; Bruscia 1981). When studies, beginning in the early 1980s, focused on ability specifically in individuals with DS, a deficit in auditory as compared to visual short-term memory was described (Marcell & Armstrong 1982; Varnhagen et al. 1987). From more recent studies in the other subcomponents of memory, a pattern of strengths and weakness associated with DS is beginning to emerge. As with many other aspects of performance, this pattern shows considerable individual variability that can, in part, be attributed to the developmental processes interacting with memory at different points in development. To fully understand its role, it is necessary to understand memory as a dynamic system, developing in concert with other cognitive and social systems, rather than a static profile of abilities.

WORKING MEMORY

AUDITORY PHONOLOGICAL LOOP

There is a consensus from studies since the early 1980s that individuals with DS have a specific deficit in the auditory/phonological loop subcomponent of working memory, resulting in poor scores in comparison with either individuals of similar developmental levels or their own performance on a variety of other cognitive tasks. Auditory phonological memory has frequently been measured with a variety of tasks such as digit span (Jarrold et al. 2002; Kay-Raining Bird & Chapman 1994; Seung & Chapman 2000; Wang & Bellugi 1994), word span (Hulme & Mackenzie 1992) and non-word repetition (Cairns & Jarrold, in press). In span tasks, digits (randomly chosen from 1 to 9) or words are presented, beginning with short sequences (usually of two words) and the length of the sequence is increased by one item after successful reproduction of the sequence until a criterion for failure is reached.

There does not now seem to be a single factor to explain an auditory working memory deficit but there are several factors that may contribute synergistically to a final outcome. The rate of articulation has been examined as a potential determiner of performance on auditory working memory tasks.

In the model of working memory proposed by Baddeley (1986) auditory information rapidly decays unless the memory trace in the phonological loop is refreshed through subvocal rehearsal. Although rehearsal may occur silently and internally, decay of the memory trace is time-dependent so the amount of information retained is determined by the rate of rehearsal and this in turn is determined, in part, by articulation rate. Individuals with DS are known to have problems in motor organisation, which includes the articulators and, thus, may be less efficient at subvocal rehearsal. However, studies addressing this issue have found weak or no relationships between the articulatory rates of adolescents and young adults with DS and their performance on verbal span tasks (Jarrold et al. 2002; Kanno & Ikeda 2002; Seung & Chapman 2000). Related to the issue of subvocal rehearsal is the question of the efficiency of the rehearsal process itself. Studies have concluded that individuals with intellectual impairment show little or no evidence of rehearsal (Hulme & Mackenzie 1992; Jarrold et al. 1999; Vicari et al. 2004). This may be related to overall developmental level, as typically developing children do not appear to use rehearsal spontaneously until seven years of age (Gathercole 1998).

A small number of studies have addressed issues related to the role of semantics and lexical access and, indirectly, the role of the episodic buffer as a support for auditory memory. When high- and low-frequency words were employed in word span tasks, adolescents with DS produced longer spans with high-frequency words, as did typically developing children of comparable mental age (MA) (Vicari et al. 2004), indicating a parallel influence of the semantic system on auditory memory. In contrast, some findings suggest that DS may be associated with difficulties in executive control of verbal material. Kanno & Ikeda (2002) observed that a semantically related word, at times, replaced the presented memory item during recall in the group with DS, suggesting difficulty in accessing temporarily stored items. When lists of words that contained semantically similar items were presented, it was found that middle-aged adults with DS made more errors than a peer group with unspecified aetiologies of MR (Kittler et al. 2004) suggesting increased susceptibility to interference and poorer executive control in verbal working memory.

In a 5 year longitudinal study nonword repetition scores at the start of the study predicted later scores on vocabulary, which could be interpreted as phonological memory having a formative role in the acquisition of vocabulary (Laws & Gunn 2004). However, in the analysis of these same data, earlier receptive vocabulary predicted later nonword repetition scores, suggesting instead a reciprocal effect.

Language ability is probably a contributing factor to performance on auditory memory span tasks, particularly when the stimuli are sentences. Sentence spans (measured in syllables) were longer than digit spans both for adolescents with DS and MA-matched controls presumably because memory was supported by familiarity with syntax (Seung & Chapman 2004).

Investigators have examined the contribution of peripheral hearing to performance on auditory memory tasks. Many individuals with DS have lifelong hearing impairments that may be undetected or untreated because they involve a mild, fluctuating hearing loss that is related to a middle-ear infections (Davies 1988). In order to determine if the auditory presentation of stimuli presents unusual difficulty for individuals with DS, testing procedures were developed to compensate for peripheral auditory impairment (Marcell & Weeks 1988; Jarrold et al. 2002). Findings indicated that while hearing levels may have some influence on performance, they do not, alone, account for the auditory memory deficits associated with DS. (The potential role of audition and auditory perception in the functioning of the phonological loop is complex. See Marcell 1995 and Jarrold et al. 2002 for a more extensive discussion of this topic.)

VISUOSPATIAL SKETCHPAD

In contrast to their difficulties with auditory verbal memory, performance on visuospatial tasks is consistent with more global measures of level-of-functioning in adolescents and adults with DS. The Corsi span task is frequently used to represent the visual system and to provide a comparison with the digit span task. In the Corsi span task, nine blocks are positioned in a random order on a board and the participant is asked to repeat the same sequence of taps as demonstrated by the tester (Milner 1971). This task, then, requires temporal and spatial sequential ability.

In general, adolescents with DS show comparable performance on the forward Corsi span to that of a peer group of individuals with MR from unspecified aetiologies (Jarrold et al. 1999) and to that of typically developing children of equivalent MA (Jarrold & Baddeley 1997).

When verbal and nonverbal spans are compared, individuals from the general population and individuals with unspecified aetiologies of MR typically show a modality effect in which auditory spans are longer than visuospatial spans (Jarrold & Baddeley 1997). However, in adolescents with DS, the spans from the two modalities are most often equal, or the visuospatial span is slightly longer (Wang & Bellugi 1994). This relationship between the two modalities, however, may not persist across the adult lifespan. Preliminary data from a study of 73 healthy adults with DS not suspected of dementia and distributed across ages 16 to 65 years indicated that performance on the Corsi span showed a faster age-associated decline than did the digit span. The different rates of change in these two domains resulted in a change in their relationship such that, by older ages, the adults with DS showed the modality effect (Figure 6.1). More importantly, adults with DS showed rapid decline during adolescence and young adulthood in an area of functioning that was a relative strength (Devenny, unpublished data).

The study of abilities dependent on the visuospatial sketchpad has recently been expanded to include more complex tasks. In a recent study (Vicari et al., in press), immediate recall of location was compared to recall of the perceptual features of geometric shapes in children and adolescents with DS and an MA-matched typically developing group of 5.2 yrs. Overall the performance of the group with DS was poorer on both visuospatial tasks but this difference between the groups was no longer significant when scores were adjusted for perceptual ability, suggesting that the basis for the relatively poorer performance by the group with DS was in part due to an impairment in perception rather than in memory.

A recent study presented five visuospatial tasks that were of progressive difficulty, requiring increasing amounts of control over working memory. It was found that while the group of adolescents with DS had similar performance to a group matched on MA for the two simplest tasks, they were significantly poorer on the two most difficult tasks (Lanfranchi et al. 2004). This study highlights the complex contribution of the central executive component of the working memory to performance on tasks and ultimately to the conclusions about relative strengths and weaknesses within and across domains. The consensus appears to be that individuals with DS have better visuospatial working memory ability than auditory phonological working memory ability and no single factor, such as articulation rate, language or hearing can entirely account for this discrepancy.

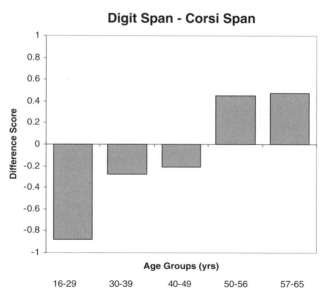

Figure 6.1. Digit span minus Corsi span for adults with DS with mild-moderate mental retardation across the adult lifespan. The numbers in each decade were: 16–29 years, N = 10; 30–39 years, N = 13; 40–49 years, N = 31; 50–55 years, N = 12; 56–65 years, N = 6.

EPISODIC MEMORY

Frequently used tasks for testing episodic memory include word-list learning and paired-associate learning in which the number of items exceeds working memory span and an individual is given several opportunities to learn the items. Although the meanings of the words used in the lists are dependent on semantic memory, the selection and juxtaposition of the words is unique to the specific testing situation and, therefore, creates conditions similar to learning associated with a specific time and place.

Compared with the many studies of working memory, there are relatively few studies that have addressed issues related to episodic memory specifically in DS when the topic was not an examination of advanced ageing. One study that compared adolescents with DS (mean age 16.7 years; mean MA 9.1 years) to a peer group with MR of unspecified aetiology and to a group of typically developing children of comparable MA, found that on a list-learning task the group with DS was poorer than both other groups (Carlesimo et al. 1997). However, when the test items were presented in a recognition paradigm the group with DS had comparable performance to the group with unspecified MR, suggesting to these investigators that DS may be associated with a deficit in the deliberate retrieval of previously stored items.

As mentioned previously, consolidation of episodic memory is associated with functioning in the hippocampus. A study comparing 28 adolescents with DS (ages 11 to 19 years) to typically developing children matched on MA (5 years of age) employed four tests that are known to be primarily dependent on hippocampal functioning. Pennington et al. (2003) found that performance of adolescents with DS was consistently poorer than the control group on each of these measures but not on other measures of executive function that are dependent on prefrontal lobe functioning. Their findings suggest that DS is associated with a specific deficit in abilities dependent on the hippocampus. It is interesting that visual as well as verbal hippocampal tasks were found to be poorer in the group with DS, a finding that contrasts with the studies of working memory. A similar finding of poorer performance by older adolescents and young adults with DS on both visual and verbal tasks of memory was also found by Vicari et al. (2000).

Episodic memory has also been tested by story recall. After the presentation of the narrative the individual is asked to retell the story. Scoring is typically the number of ideas from the original story that are reproduced. Clearly, the ability to perform well on this task is related to language competence in addition to memory ability. After watching a wordless 6 minute film, *The Pear Story*, children with DS were asked to recount the events they had seen (Boudreau & Chapman 2000). Children with DS were better able to recount the event structure than a comparison group of typically developing children with the same level of expressive language (as measured by mean length of utterance) and were similar to typically developing children with comparable comprehension. In contrast, when a short story was presented auditorily, recall was very much poorer in individuals with DS (score = 0.6, maximum possible score = 8) as compared to those with the unspecified MR (3.4) or typically developing children (5.2) (Carlisimo et al. 1997).

Episodic memory is vulnerable to changes associated with normal ageing processes and its decline is one of the earliest signs of dementia of the Alzheimer-type (DAT). Even though the effects of ageing on the memory system are imposed on an organisation that has an atypical developmental history in adults with DS, findings show a pattern of performance similar to that seen in the general population. Small age-related declines in episodic memory have been shown in longitudinal studies of healthy older adults with DS but they occur precociously, almost 20 years earlier than in the general population (Haxby & Schapiro, 1992; Devenny et al. 1996, 2002; Oliver et al. 1998; Krinsky-McHale et al. 2002).

The distinction between memory declines related to normal ageing and those related to DAT is particularly important in adults with DS because they are uniquely vulnerable to Alzheimer's disease. Virtually all adults with DS develop the neuropathological hallmarks of this disease (neurofibrillary tangles, amyloid plaques and neural cell loss) with the deposition of amyloid beginning in their third decade of life (Hof et al. 1995; Hyman et al. 1995; see Mann 1993 for a review). However, only some individuals develop the symptoms of dementia and, typically, not until more than 20 years later. A decline in episodic memory is an early symptom associated with DAT in individuals with DS (and in the general population) and is distinguished from decline associated with normal ageing by the degree and type of memory impairment (Devenny et al. 2002; Krinsky-McHale et al. 2002). In one study we asked older adults with DS to learn a list of 12 unrelated words along with a unique category identifier. For those who were healthy, presenting the category cue substantially improved their recall of test items. For those adults who subsequently developed dementia sometime within the following four years, the category cue was much less effective in facilitating their recall (Devenny et al. 2002).

Individuals with DS appear to have more difficulty with tasks of episodic memory than their peers with MR from other aetiologies or typically developing children of comparable MA. Unlike working memory individuals with DS show relative impairments on tasks of visuospatial as well as verbal episodic memory.

SEMANTIC MEMORY

The ability to acquire and retain new vocabulary reflects the integrity of semantic memory. In general, children, adolescents and adults with DS have comprehension vocabularies commensurate with their overall level of functioning, and vocabulary is maintained or may even increase through later adult life as the result of exposure to new activities. Individuals with DS are sensitive to semantic categories as shown by their ability to use category cues to enhance recall of word lists (Devenny et al. 2002). On our version of the Selective Reminding Test, a list-learning task in which all the items are from a single semantic category (animals or foods), we have observed that when intrusions of words that were not on the list occur, they are most often from the same semantic category. In another study, however, even with facility with semantic categories, adolescents with DS, did not make effective use of category information in order to support free recall (Carlesimo et al. 1997).

IMPLICIT MEMORY

There have been very few studies examining implicit memory specifically in individuals with DS, and only one in which multiple subcomponents of implicit memory were tested within the same study (Vicari et al. 2000). The performance of adolescents and young adults was compared to that of typically developing children of similar MA (6.3 years) on two procedural learning tasks: the Tower of London and a Serial Reaction Time Test, and two repetition priming tasks, the Fragmented Picture Test and Stem Completion. The performance of the groups was comparable on the procedural learning tasks and both groups showed evidence of priming. In contrast, on measures of explicit memory in this study, the group with DS showed poorer performance.

One of the properties of implicit memory is its insensitivity to age and IQ relative to explicit memory. In a recent study middle-aged and older adults with DS (mean age = 44.4 + 6 years; mean IQ = 59 + 6.8) were compared to adults with Williams syndrome and to adults with MR from unspecified aetiologies of similar ages and levels of functioning (Krinsky-McHale et al., 2005). Implicit memory was measured by the Fragmented Pictures Task while explicit memory was measured by the Selective Reminding Test. A direct comparison of performance on these measures indicated age-associated declines on explicit memory only for the groups with DS and Williams syndrome; no declines on implicit memory for any of the three groups were found.

Implicit memory in individuals with DS appears to be consistent with their level of functioning and to be relatively resistant to age-associated changes.

COMPARISON WITH OTHER AETIOLOGY GROUPS

At present it is not certain whether the pattern of strengths and weaknesses in memory ability described by the studies of individuals with DS is unique to this syndrome. With the possible exception of Williams syndrome there is not enough information about ability across all the components of memory to describe profiles for other genetic causes of MR. Also, with few exceptions (for example, Wang & Bellugi 1994; Klein & Mervis 1999; Munir et al. 2000; Jarrold et al. 2004; Vicari et al., in press), studies typically examine performance in only a single syndrome and often only a single component of memory, making it difficult to infer a broad pattern of abilities. Given the diverse developmental trajectories associated with various genetic syndromes, it seems likely that many of these syndromes will eventually be associated with specific behavioural phenotypes.

Our understanding of the pattern of strengths and weaknesses associated with Williams syndrome is changing, as recent research has shown a complex profile of abilities. In general, their visuospatial working memory, particularly when processing involves memory for spatial location, is relatively poor (Vicari 2001; see Farran & Jarrold 2003 for review) when compared to their verbal working memory. This weakness in visual processing is also found in tasks dependent on long-term memory where, again, spatial location memory is poorer than memory for the visual memory for the details of objects (Vicari et al. 2005). Preliminary evidence of age-associated declines in episodic memory indicating premature ageing similar to DS were found in a small group of adults with WS (Devenny et al. 2004; Krinsky-McHale et al., 2005). With regard to implicit memory, priming appears to be consistent with overall level-of-functioning (Vicari 2001) and is not disrupted by ageing (Krinsky-McHale et al., in press) while procedural learning appears to be poorer in adolescents and adults with Williams syndrome than in typically developing individuals (Vicari 2001; Don et al. 2003).

In general, the strengths and weaknesses of memory abilities in DS and in Williams syndrome reflect a broader pattern of cognitive abilities. Individuals with DS are known to have difficulty with verbal ability and expressive language in particular (Chapman & Hesketh 2000). For individuals with Williams syndrome, verbal ability is an area of relative strength but visuospatial abilities are compromised (Farran & Jarrold 2003). It is likely that future studies of the interaction of memory with other cognitive abilities will reveal that the direction of influence will depend on the developmental age of individuals. For example, whereas auditory and phonological abilities may be a strong influence on early vocabulary and language development in very young children (Gathercole 1998), for older children and adolescents language ability may determine verbal memory ability.

CONCLUSIONS

Memory ability in individuals with DS has a characteristic pattern of strengths and weaknesses across the various sub-components of the memory system. Auditory working memory appears to be selectively compromised during childhood, adolescence and young adulthood, as is episodic memory. Memory that is based on semantic knowledge and implicit learning, however, is consistent with individual overall levels of functioning. It is this pattern of abilities that may be specific to DS, not ability related to any single subcomponent of memory. However, to some extent, this pattern of memory abilities is determined by the design of research studies and is strongly influenced by the composition and age of the comparison group. (For discussion of the influence of matching variables on performance outcomes across comparison groups see Jarrold & Baddeley 1997; Chapman & Hesketh 2000; Vicari & Carlesimo 2002; Farran & Jarrold 2003.)

Although a pattern of strengths and weaknesses associated with DS seems to exist, there is also considerable individual variability.

Stating that a particular pattern of memory abilities is the behavioural outcome associated with DS does not address the aetiology of that particular pattern. Extrapolating from the very few studies of infants with DS, early memory ability does not conform to the observed behavioural phenotype in later life (Paterson et al. 1999). It appears that the pattern of memory abilities described for adolescents and young adults may be an emergent phenomenon, linked, perhaps, to differential rates and trajectories of development within the subcomponents of the memory system. If a behavioural phenotype for memory processes associated with DS emerges, it exists for a circumscribed duration because the processes of ageing that alter specific memory abilities begin in the early adult years in this population.

Memory is a fundamental process that contributes to the development of other domains such as cognition, language, social skills and affect, just as it is influenced by all the other processes that develop in concert with it. It would be helpful if future studies included memory in the context of everyday experiences, such as flashbulb memory (the memory for scarce and emotionally charged events), eyewitness memory, false memory, prospective memory (memory for actions to be taken in the future), face memory and autobiographical memory (the selection, retention, and manipulation of the memory of life events). Thus far, studies of memory have been almost exclusively confined to the visual and auditory modalities. Future studies associated with other sensory functions, including olfaction, taction and kinaesthesia, will promote a more complete understanding of memory in this population.

Although considerable progress has been made since the mid-1980s in describing memory processes associated with DS, as yet we do not know which factors related to memory abilities are most amenable to intervention, at what age intervention should occur or whether the intervention should be targeted or nonspecific. Just how intervention in another domain, such as language, will influence memory development remains to be determined. We do know, however, that memory is sensitive to development and this suggests that interventions that promote successful development will likely have a significant impact on memory.

ACKNOWLEDGEMENTS

This research was supported in part by funds from the New York State Office of Mental Retardation and Developmental Disabilities and by NIH grants RO1 AG 14771 to D. A. Devenny and PO1 HD35897 to W. Silverman. The author wishes to thank S. J. Krinsky-McHale, P. Kittler and C. Marino for their many and substantive contributions to the research conducted in the Lifespan Development Laboratory and to W. Silverman for his continued support.

REFERENCES

Baddeley, A. D. (1986) *Working Memory*. Oxford: Clarendon Press.
Baddeley, A. D. (2000) The episodic buffer: a new component of working memory? *Trends Cognit Sci*, **4**, 417–423.
Baddeley, A. D. (2001) Is working memory still working? *Am Psychol*, **56**, 851–864.
Belmont, J. M. (1966) Long-term memory in mental retardation. In N. R. Ellis (ed.) *Int Rev Res Ment Retard*. New York: Academic Press, pp. 219–255.
Boudreau, D., Chapman, R. S. (2000) The relationship between event representation and linguistic skill in narratives of children and adolescents with Down syndrome. *Journal of Speech, Language, and Hearing Research*, **43**, 1146–1159.
Bruscia, K. E. (1981) Auditory short–term memory and attentional control of mentally retarded persons. *Am J Ment Def*, **85**, 435–437.
Cairns, P., Jarrold, C. (in press) Exploring the correlates of impaired nonword repetition in Down syndrome. *Br J Dev Psychol*.
Carlesimo, G. A., Marotta, L., Vicari, S. (1997) Long-term memory in mental retardation: evidence for a specific impairment in subjects with Down's syndrome. *Neuropsychologia*, **35**, 71–79.
Chapman, R. S., Hesketh, L. (2000) The behavioral phenotype of Down syndrome. *Mental Retardation and Developmental Disabilities Research Review*, **6**, 84–95.
Davies, B. (1988) Auditory disorders in Down's syndrome. *Scand Audiol, Suppl*, **30**, 65–68.
Devenny, D. A., Krinsky–McHale, S. J., Kittler, P. M., Flory, M., Jenkins, E., Brown, W. T. (2004) Age–associated memory changes in adults with Williams syndrome. *Dev Neuropsychol*, **26**, 691–706.
Devenny, D. A., Silverman, W. P., Hill, A. L., Jenkins, E., Sersen, E. A., Wisniewski, K. E. (1996) Normal aging in adults with Down syndrome: a longitudinal study. *J Intellect Disabil Res*, **40**, 208–221.
Devenny, D. A., Zimmerli, E. J., Kittler, P., Krinsky-McHale, S. J. (2002) Cued recall in early-stage dementia in adults with Down syndrome. *J Intellect Disabil Res*, **46**, 472–483.
Don, A. J., Schellenberg, E. G., Reber, A. S., DiGirolamo, K. M., Wang, P. P. (2003) Implicit learning in children and adults with Williams syndrome. *Dev Neuropsychol*, **23**, 201–225.
Ellis, N. R. (1970) Memory processes in retardates and normals. In N. R. Ellis (ed.) *International Review of Research on Mental Retardation*. New York: Academic Press, pp. 1–32.

Ellis, N. R., McCarver, R. B., Ashurst, Jr., H. M. (1970) Short-term memory in the retarded: ability level and stimulus meaningfulness. *Am J Ment Retard*, **75**, 72–80.

Farran, E. K., Jarrold, C. (2003) Visuospatial cognition in Williams Syndrome: reviewing and accounting for the strengths and weaknesses in performance. *Dev Neuropsychol*, **23**, 172–200.

Gathercole, S. E. (1998) The development of memory. *J Child Psychol Psychiatr*, **39**, 3–27.

Gibson, D. (1978) *Down's Syndrome: The Psychology of Mongolism*. Cambridge: Cambridge University Press.

Graf, P., Schacter, D. L. (1985) Implicit and explicit memory for new associations in normal and amnestic subjects. *J Exp Psychol Learn Mem Cognit*, **11**, 501–518.

Haxby, J. V., Schapiro, M. D. (1992) Longitudinal study of neuropsychological function in older adults with Down syndrome. In L. Nadel, C. J. Epstein (eds) *Down Syndrome and Alzheimer Disease*. New York: Wiley-Liss, pp. 35–50.

Hof, P. R., Bouras, C., Perl, D. P., Sparks, I., Mehta, N., Morrison, J. H. (1995) Age–related distribution of neuropathologic changes in the cerebral cortex of patients with Down's syndrome. *Arch Neurol*, **52**, 379–391.

Hulme, C., Mackenzie, S. (1992) *Working Memory and Severe Learning Difficulties*. Hillsdale NJ: Lawrence Erlbaum.

Hyman, B. T., West, H. L., Rebeck, G. W., Lai, F., Mann, D. M. A. (1995) Neuro-pathological changes in Down's syndrome hippocampal formation. *Archives of Neurology*, **52**, 373–378.

Jarrold, C., Baddeley, A. D. (1997) Short-term memory for verbal and visuospatial information in Down's syndrome. *Cognitive Neuropsychiatry*, **2**, 101–122.

Jarrold, C., Baddeley, A. D., Hewes, A. K. (1999) Genetically dissociated components of working memory: evidence from Down's and Williams' syndrome. *Neuropsychologia*, **37**, 637–651.

Jarrold, C., Baddeley, A., Phillips, C. E. (2002) Verbal short-term memory in Down syndrome: a problem of memory, audition, or speech? *Journal of Speech, Language, and Hearing Research*, **45**, 531–544.

Jarrold, C., Cowan, N., Hewes, A. K., Riby, D. M. (2004) Speech timing and verbal short-term memory: evidence for contrasting deficits in Down syndrome and Williams syndrome. *J Mem Lang*, **51**, 365–380.

Kanno, K., Ikeda, Y. (2002) Word-length effect in verbal short-term memory in individuals with Down's syndrome. *J Intellect Disabil Res*, **46**, 613–618.

Kay-Raining Bird, E., Chapman, R. S. (1994) Sequential recall in individuals with Down syndrome. *Journal of Speech and Hearing Research*, **37**, 1369–1380.

Kittler, P., Krinsky-McHale, S. J., Devenny, D. A. (2004) Semantic and phonological loop effects on verbal working memory in middle-aged adults with mental retardation. *Am J Ment Retard*, **109**, 467–480.

Klein, B. P., Mervis, C. B. (1999) Cognitive strengths and weaknesses of 9- and 10-year-olds with Williams syndrome or Down syndrome. *Dev Neuropsychol*, **16**, 177–196.

Krinsky-McHale, S. J., Devenny, D. A., Kittler, P., Silverman, W. (2003) Implicit memory in aging adults with mental retardation with and without Down syndrome. *Am J Ment Retard*, **108**, 219–233.

Krinsky-McHale, S. J., Devenny, D. A., Silverman, W. P. (2002) Changes in explicit memory associated with early dementia in adults with Down's syndrome. *J Intellect Disabil Res*, **46**, 198–208.

Krinsky-McHale, S. J., Kittler, P., Brown, W. T., Jenkins, E. C., Devenny, D. A. (2005) Repetition priming in adults with Williams syndrome: an age-related dissociation between implicit and explicit memory. *Am J Ment Retard,* **110**, 482–496.

Lanfranchi, S., Cornoldi, C., Vianello, R. (2004) Verbal and visuospatial working memory deficits in children with Down syndrome. *Am J Ment Retard*, **109**, 456–466.

Laws, G., Gunn, D. (2004) Phonological memory as a predictor of language comprehension in Down syndrome: a five-year follow-up study. *J Child Psychol Psychiatr*, **45**, 326–337.

Mann, D. M. A. (1993) Association between Alzheimer disease and Down syndrome: neuropathological observations. In J. M. Berg, K. Karlinsky, A. J. Holland (eds) *Alzheimer Disease, Down Syndrome, and their Relationship.* Oxford: Oxford University Press, pp. 711–792.

Marcell, M. M. (1995) Relationships between hearing and auditory cognition in Down's syndrome youth. *Down's Syndrome: Research and Practice*, **3**, 75–91.

Marcell, M. M., Armstrong, J. (1982) Auditory and visual sequential memory of Down's syndrome and nonretarded children. *Am J Ment Defic*, **87**, 86–95.

Marcell, M. M., Weeks, S. L. (1988) Short-term memory difficulties and Down's syndrome. *J Ment Def Res*, **32**, 153–162.

Milner, B. (1971) Interhemispheric differences in the localization of psychological processes in man. *Br Med Bull*, **3**, 272–277.

Munir, F., Cornish, K. M., Wilding, J. (2000) Nature of the working memory deficit in fragile–X syndrome. *Brain Cognit*, **44**, 387–401.

Oliver, C., Crayton, L., Holland, A., Hall, S., Bradbury, J. (1998) A four year prospective study of age-related cognitive change in adults with Down syndrome. *Psychol Med*, **28**, 1365–1377.

Paterson, S. J., Brown, J. H., Gsödl, M. K., Johnson, M. H., Karmiloff–Smith, A. (1999) Cognitive modularity and genetic disorders. *Science*, **286**, 2355–2358.

Pennington, B. F., Moon, J., Edgin, J., Stedron, J., Nadel, L. (2003) The neuropsychology of Down syndrome: evidence for hippocampal dysfunction. *Child Dev*, **74**, 75–93.

Schacter, D. L. (1987) Implicit memory: history and current status. *Journal of Experimental Psychology: Learning, Memory, and Cognition*, **13**, 501–518.

Schacter, D. L., Tulving, E. (1994) *Memory Systems.* Cambridge: MIT Press.

Seung, H.-K., Chapman, R. (2000) Digit span in individuals with Down syndrome and in typically developing children: temporal aspects. *Journal of Speech, Language, and Hearing Research*, **43**, 609–620.

Seung, H.-K., Chapman, R. (2004) Sentence memory of individuals with Down's syndrome and typically developing children. *Journal of Intellectual Disability Research*, **48**, 160–171.

Squire, L. R. (1987) *Memory and Brain.* New York: Oxford University Press.

Tulving, E. (1983) *Elements of Episodic Memory.* Oxford: Claredon.

Tulving, E. (2002) Episodic memory: from mind to brain. *Annu Rev Psychol*, **53**, 1–25.

Varnhagen, C. K., Das, J. P., Varnhagen, S. (1987) Auditory and visual memory span: cognitive processing by TMR individuals with Down syndrome and other etiologies. *Am J Ment Defic*, **91**, 398–405.

Vicari, S. (2001) Implicit versus explicit memory function in children with Down and Williams syndrome. *Down Syndrome Research and Practice*, **7**, 35–40.

Vicari, S., Bellucci, S., Carlesimo, G. A. (2000) Implicit and explicit memory: a functional dissociation in persons with Down syndrome. *Neuropsychologia*, **38**, 240–251.

Vicari, S., Bellucci, S., Carlesimo, G. A. (2005) Visual and spatial long-term memory: differential pattern of impairments in Williams and Down syndromes. *Dev Med Child Neurol*, **47**, 305–311.

Vicari, S., Bellucci, S., Carlesimo, G. A. (in press) Evidence from two genetic syndromes for independence of spatial and visual working memory. *Dev Med Child Neurol*.

Vicari, S., Marotta, L., Carlesimo, G. A. (2004) Verbal short-term memory in Down's syndrome: an articulatory loop deficit? *J Intellect Disabil Res*, **48**, 80–92.

Wang, P. P., Bellugi, U. (1994) Evidence from two genetic syndromes for a dissociation between verbal and visual-spatial short-term memory. *J Clin Exp Neuropsychol*, **16**, 317–322.

Wang, P. P., Doherty, S., Rourke, S. B., Bellugi, U. (1995) Unique profile of visuoperceptual skills in a genetic syndrome. *Brain Cognit*, **29**, 54–65.

7 Specific Language Profiles in Down Syndrome and Other Genetic Syndromes of Mental Retardation

JEAN-ADOLPHE RONDAL
University of Liege, Belgium
University of Udine, Italy

SUMMARY

Major aspects of language development and functioning in Down syndrome (DS) as well as other genetic syndromes associated with mental retardation are analysed with the aim of establishing whether this field supplies arguments in favour of a specificity hypothesis regarding the language phenotype in individuals with DS. It is concluded that a number of indications exist that can be interpreted as favouring syndromic specificity, not in the sense of individual pathognomonic features but in showing a particular profile of relative strengths and weaknesses among language components. It is further suggested that each genetic syndrome associated with mental retardation may have its specific profile. These profiles find their sources in the particular genotypes and neurological phenotypes characterising each syndrome.

INTRODUCTION

There are several hundred genetic syndromes that lead to mental retardation (MR). Shprintzen (1997) lists more than 200 genetic conditions conducive to language, speech and communication disorders. His list includes a large number of MR syndromes. Mental retardation of genetic origin represents 30% of all cases of moderate and severe retardation and 15% of all cases of mild MR. Given current knowledge concerning a number of genetic syndromes involving MR (Hodapp et al. 2000; Rondal et al. 2004) the issue of the relative specificity of the major neurobehavioural features of these syndromes is relevant. Until recently it was thought that the key dimension in MR was the level of mental functioning estimated by intelligence quotient

Down Syndrome: Neurobehavioural Specificity. Edited by JA Rondal and J Perera.
© 2006 John Wiley & Sons Ltd.

(IQ), together with an estimate of adaptive potential. This view, although relevant, remains too general. The scientific approach to MR needs to take the aetiological dimension into account more. For theoretical and clinical reasons we must establish, on a firmer basis, which neurobehavioural features differ from one entity to another, to what extent and which features are found within several or all the MR syndromes to a comparable extent.

Specificity (the property of something that has particular characteristics or a property pertaining characteristically to an entity) can be envisaged at two levels:

- the level of individual features or symptoms
- a systemic level that takes into account the relationships between these features and symptoms (Rondal 1995)

The first relates to the concept of pathognomony – a feature belonging exclusively to a nosological category – hence the diagnosis. It is not clear at the present time that nonaetiological pathognomonic features exist in Down syndrome (DS). Even the chromosomic nondisjunction and other aberrations aetiologically related to the condition are common in MR of genetic origin (Shprintzen 1997). Pathognomonic features in MR syndromes are extremely rare. Cases include compulsive overeating, found only (as a generic feature) in Prader-Willi syndrome (Dykens et al. 2000) or failure of locomotion in late infancy in Rett syndrome (Segawa 2001).

Research has uncovered a large number of symptomatic features in DS that, taken together, yield a specific picture of the syndrome (some authors have used the expression 'partial specificity' – for example, Dykens et al. 2000). This amounts to changing the notion of syndrome (usually defined as the set of symptoms characteristic of a pathological entity) with no requirement that any constituting feature be pathognomonic or even restricted to a limited number of entities. The issue must be dealt with taking into account the whole spectrum of neurobehavioural and personality characteristics, health, and degenerative susceptibility with ageing, as well as the possible indirect effects of the above on affective and sexual development, family and peer relationships, school, social and professional inclusion.

Intersyndromic comparison is a key methodological tool, for one cannot talk of peculiarities in any syndrome without making a systematic comparison with other entities (Rondal et al. 2004; Mervis & Robinson 2005). Without prejudging the ultimate answer that will be given to the specificity question (whether or not to reject the 'null hypothesis') it is relevant to list a number of empirical indications that seem to corroborate the specificity claim. This is the objective of the present book. The practical implications of this trend of research are most important because reasoned therapeutic and rehabilitation policies depend on precisely defining what is specific and what is more general in the MR syndrome phenotypes. The idea is that specific aspects call for particular intervention approaches tailored to the particular needs of people with given syndromes, and nonspecific aspects require more general approaches extending across a diversity of nosologic entities.

In what follows I shall concentrate on speech and language, referring to the major language components (phonology, lexicon, semantics, morphosyntax, pragmatics, and discourse). The specificity question will be addressed through a comparison of language development and functioning in several MR syndromes of genetic origin.

DOWN SYNDROME (DS)

Down syndrome is the most common nonherited chromosomal MR condition, with a prevalence close to 1 in 1000 of live births. Aetiologically, DS is due to an increased number of gene copies (gene dosage) in some or all of the 225 genes composing the DNA (deoxyribonucleic acid) sequence for chromosome 21 (Capone 2001).

No major language differences have been demonstrated between the three main aetiological subcategories of DS (standard trisomy 21, accounting for 97% of the cases; translocations, accounting for 2%; and mosaïcism, 1%; in these latter cases the embryos develop with a mosaic of normal and trisomic cells) except for a possible slight referential lexical superiority of mosaic DS subjects, who tend to have higher IQs (Fishler & Koch 1991).

Prelinguistic development shows significant delays in DS infants. Turn-taking skills, basic for future conversational exchanges, are slow to develop. The type of prelinguistic phrasing that can be observed in typically developing (TD) babies, beginning around 3 months of age (intermittent babbling, approximately 3 seconds long, with phrase-ending syllables lasting longer than other syllables) is different in DS babies. They take longer to finish a phrase. The sounds of babbling are mostly similar in types and tokens in TD and DS infants (Smith & Oller 1981). Articulatory development is slow and difficult in the latter. In the most serious cases (with markedly reduced speech intelligibility) one may suspect developmental apraxia (Kumin 2001) or (better) dyspraxia of speech. The overall speech progression, however, parallels that of TD children, even if many DS children exhibit more inconsistent segmental development (Dodd & Leahy 1989).

Many DS children do not demonstrate consistent production of conventional words before 2 or 3 years chronological age (CA). Their shortcomings in motor development (Wishart 1988) favour the delays. The articulatory difficulties also contribute to lexical retardation. Semantic development is delayed in DS in proportion to the general cognitive impairment characteristic of the condition. Early lexical development (both productive and receptive) generally shows a positive linear relation with mental age (MA) increase (Rondal & Edwards 1997). However, the rate of DS children's acquisition of new words does not keep up with that of TD children and the equations describing both vocabulary learning curves gradually differ more and more as to slope (Miller 1999). The gap continues to widen with increasing CA, particularly for productive lexicon (Cardoso-Martins et al. 1985).

The first multiword productions are often observed around 3 or 4 years CA in DS children. When they begin to combine two and three words within the same utterance, DS children appear to express the same range of relational meanings or thematic roles and relations as reported by the students of early combinatorial language in TD children. These relate to the semantic structures of the natural languages. Examples of early thematic relations expressed by MR, as well as by TD children, are notice of existence, denial, disappearance, recurrence, attribution, possession, location, instrument, conjunction, agent-action, action-object and agent-action.

Mean length of utterance (MLU) is widely used as a criterion variable for assessing language development. Up to a certain level of development each morphosyntactic acquisition is directly reflected in the MLU count. Mean length of utterance development in DS shows a good linear relationship with CA until early adolescence (Rondal & Comblain 1996). Mean length of utterance values of 1 are usually observed around 2 years. Between 2 and 9 or 10 years, MLU goes from values of 1 to 4 approximately. Mean lengths of utterance of 5 or 6 units are often observed from 12 years. TD children reach MLU levels of 5 units and more around 6 years. In conversational speech between TD adults, the average MLU values are close to 12. The slowness and limitation of MLU development in DS correspond to lasting shortcomings in morphosyntax. Productive use of grammatical words (articles, prepositions, pronouns, conjunctions, auxiliaries) and morphological marking of gender, number, tense, mode and aspect are limited (O'Neill & Henry 2002). Word order in those languages relying on strict sequential devices to express thematic relations (for example, English and French) is usually correct (Rondal 1978; Rosenberg & Abbeduto 1993).

Numerous reports point to serious limitations of DS children and adolescents in the comprehension of morphosyntactic structures and their lagging behind MA-matched TD controls in this respect (Rondal & Edwards 1997).

Young DS children (1 to 4 years) use one-word utterances to request objects located out of reach (Greenwald & Leonard 1979). Few differences exist between MA-matched or MLU-matched TD and DS children in the frequency of speech acts, for example question-answer, assertion, suggestion, request, command (Coggins et al. 1983). Preschoolers with DS and TD toddlers matched for expressive language make the greatest use of the 'answering' speech act when interacting with their mothers (Owens & MacDonald 1982). The turn-taking behaviour of DS adolescents is mostly rule governed and systematic. Limitations are observed, however, in the use of linguistic forms that TD people find appropriate for the expression of particular speech acts.

A study by Boudreau & Chapman (2000) on linguistic expression of event representation in narratives suggests that DS adolescents and young adults deal with event structures in narratives in the same way as MA-matched TD children. Regarding use of linguistic devices and cohesion, however, DS individuals perform more poorly than MA-matched controls. Other works (Reilly et al. 1990; Chapman et al. 1991) confirm the particular difficulty of DS children and adolescents in various aspects of online storytelling and processing. Despite expressive lexical and syntactic limitations, adolescents and young adults with DS are able to express more narrative content and develop higher level story schemas than MLU-matched TD controls (Miles & Chapman 2002), which could be the result of the DS subjects' longer experience with listening to stories.

The speech and language of people with DS can be best defined in generic terms as presenting marked phonological and morphosyntactic deficiencies in conjunction with relatively preserved semantic and pragmatic dispositions. I shall not discuss the noticeable and at times marked interindividual differences existing in the language abilities of DS individuals (cf. Rondal 1995, 2003). Such a variability raises interesting theoretical questions and should be taken into account clinically, but does not contradict the general pattern discussed here.

WILLIAMS SYNDROME (WS)

This is a congenital metabolic disorder (prevalence: one case in approximately 25 000 births – Martin et al. 1984). The condition is associated with hemizygous deletion (concerning only one chromosome in the pair) of a set of genes (18 identified so far) including the elastin locus at 7q11.23 (Korenberg et al. 2000).

Globally, language ability is a relative strength for individuals with WS (Mervis et al. 2003). Indeed, WS and DS are almost opposites in terms of their strengths and weaknesses.

Many adolescents and adults with WS have good referential lexical abilities (Bellugi et al. 1990). Early vocabulary development is usually as delayed in WS as it is in DS (Bellugi et al. 2000) but later things improve considerably for most WS subjects. Vocabulary scores of many adolescents and young adults with WS are closer to their CAs than their MAs (Bellugi et al. 1988). The relatively high vocabulary scores displayed by many WS individuals in lexical tasks do not necessarily reflect a normal development pathway, however. Stevens & Karmiloff-Smith (1997) compared a WS group and a TD MA-matched control group in the range of CA 3–9 years for processing constraints on word learning. As argued in the literature (for example, Markman 1990), in construing the meaning of new words TD children display an understanding of mutual exclusivity (an object cannot have more than one name), whole objects (a novel word heard in the presence of a novel object refers to the whole object rather than to its substance, properties, or component features) and taxonomic constraints (lexical categories are constituted of entities or events of the same types as opposed, for example, to thematic or linear associations. Whereas WS children show fast mapping and mutual exclusivity, they do not seem to abide by the whole object and taxonomic constraints. This suggests that despite sometimes advanced vocabulary ages, the processes underlying lexical acquisition and organisation in semantic memory may follow a path somewhat different from that of TD individuals (see also Nazzi & Karmiloff-Smith 2002; Nazzi et al. 2003). It is, of course, tempting to relate the apparent absence of the whole object constraint in the lexical learning of WS children to their serious difficulties in visuospatial integration (Stiles et al. 2000).

Speech in WS is usually fluent with correct articulation and prosody. The voice may be hoarse. Sentence comprehension and use of morphosyntactic devices are not intact (Capirci et al. 1996; Bellugi et al. 2000), contrary to early suggestions, even if globally the productive syntax of many WS subjects appears relatively advanced (see also Volterra et al. 2003). Careful scrutiny (Thomas et al. 2001) reveals that WS subjects are CA delayed (but not MA delayed, or much less MA delayed) in the acquisition of past-tense forms in English (irregular forms being worse than regular ones).

Discursive ability is relatively preserved in WS. Reilly et al. (1990) compared cognitively matched WS and DS adolescents in a storytelling task. In contrast to DS subjects, the WS adolescents told cohesive and complex narrative making good use of affective prosody. Pragmatics is the area of major weakness in WS. These individuals have difficulties with topic introduction, topic maintenance, turn taking and in maintaining appropriate eye contact in dyadic face-to-face interactions. Their speech is often odd, socially inappropriate, and repetitive with incessant questions. At times they may echo the interlocutor's utterances with apparent limited understanding (Volterra et al. 1994).

FRAGILE-X SYNDROME (FXS)

This is an X-linked disorder passed on through generations. It is the leading inherited cause of MR with a prevalence of 1 in 4000 males (Turner et al. 1996). Surveys (for example, Webb et al. 1986) show that FXS accounts for 2% of MR among males. The cytogenetic expression of the fragile site is Xq27.3. It is caused by a trinucleotide repeat mutation, which is associated with methylation and resultant transcriptional silencing of the FMR gene (Verkerk et al. 1991). The expression of FMR protein varies substantially between cases with either mosaicism, either partially methylated or fully methylated. This variation accounts for a small but significant proportion of variance in levels of early motor, social, adaptive, cognitive and language development in males with FXS (Bailey et al. 2001). Twenty per cent of males with the errant gene present no pathological symptom (are nonpenetrant). The rest of the affected males are moderately to severely mentally retarded (Maes et al. 1994). Approximately one-third of the females are affected with a phenotypic variant of the syndrome determining learning difficulties. A minority is impaired with mild to moderate MR (Hagerman 1996). These females have inherited FX from a carrier mother. Premutation carriers have trinucleotide repeats in the 50 to 200 range whereas individuals with a full mutation have more than 200 repeats (Pennington 1995).

The language picture for the males affected with FXS is summarised as follows. Speech tends to be fast, perseverative, with fluctuating rates, increased loudness, and sometimes oral apraxia (Wolf-Schein et al. 1987). Unusual voice effect, dysrhythmia, echolalia, speech impulsiveness, disrupted prosody, and poor intelligibility, have been noted (Borgraef et al. 1987). However, dysfluencies in males with FXS differ from developmental stuttering on several aspects, for example, dominating once-only repetitions, function words more affected than content ones, and between-word dysfluencies more frequent than within-word dysfluencies (Van Borsel et al. 2005). Some FXS children speak with a high-pitched voice. They frequently omit or substitute vocalic or consonant phonemes (Vilkman et al. 1988). Receptive vocabulary is relatively preserved (Gérard et al. 1997). However, word-finding difficulties have been reported (Spinelli et al. 1995). Utterance formulation is restricted and productive morphosyntax deficient (Sudhalter et al. 1991). Receptive language is also deficient and slow to develop but less so than expressive language (Roberts et al. 2001). The language of FXS subjects is pragmatically limited with poor topic maintenance and turn-taking difficulties (Abbeduto & Hagerman 1997). Discourse is poorly constructed and lacks cohesion (Sudhalter et al. 1991). The corresponding state of affairs for the affected and the carrier females is still less clear (see Murphy & Abbeduto 2003, however, for an initial summary of data).

Languagewise, males with FXS stand somewhat in between DS and WS individuals. They show relatively preserved lexical and morphosyntactic abilities together with limited pragmatical abilities like WS persons. They also present marked speech difficulties, which are not of the same type as those found in DS. Fragile X syndrome males' difficulties have more to do with a lack of fluency than with the realisation of the articulatory units, as is typically the case in DS. The same language components may be affected in different genetic syndromes involving MR, but to differing extents and as a result of different processes and mechanisms.

The language characteristics of a limited number of other genetic syndromes have begun to be studied (cf. Rondal 2004; Rondal & Comblain, in press; for further analyses). Some syndromes appear to be gravely detrimental to language development.

RETT SYNDROME (RS)

This is peculiar because it is a progressive disorder. It affects 1 in 10000 to 15000 individuals. Mutations in the gene MECP2 at Xq28, 2 seem to be the major cause of this linked dominant neurodevelopmental disorder, occurring almost exclusively in females (Xiang et al. 2000). The mutations are found in 100% of the patients with classic RS. Their prevalence in atypical RS (preserved-speech-variant type-PSV) is still uncertain (Auranen et al. 2001) but they could relate in major ways to the MECP2 gene as well (Yamashita et al. 2001).

Most infants with RS develop within expected limits until approximately 6 to 12 months of age (Kerr & Corbitt 1994; Dunn 2001). Regression occurs (between 1 and 3 years) drastically affecting language, motor, and cognitive acquisitions. By 7 years of age, RS children are severely intellectually disabled (Witt-Engerstrom 1987). In many RS children (with the classic Rett syndrome), language rarely develops beyond prelinguistic acquisition and single words. In some cases there is a complete failure to develop language (alalia – Trevathan & Moser 1988); subjects do not even show behaviours interpretable as elementary intentions to communicate (for example, joint attention, gaze shifts, and turns). However, some RS girls (around 5%) (of the PSV-type) keep an ability to use at least some grammatical language produced with articulation difficulties (Zappella 1997).

PRADER-WILLI SYNDROME (PWS)

This has a prevalence of 1 in 10000 to 1 in 15000 births (Cassidy 1997) or 1 in 15000 to 1 in 30000, equally affecting both sexes (Daniel & Gridley 1998). About 70% of cases are associated with a silencing (technically labelled genomic imprinting when one of the two allele genes is silenced whereas the other is expressed) of a number (not yet defined with precision) of genes on the chromosome 15 (region q11-13) of maternal origin together with the simultaneous deletion of the same part of the chromosome 15 of paternal origin (Butler et al. 1986). As a consequence, the maternal alleles cannot compensate for the deleted paternal genes given that they have been silenced (Everman & Cassidy 2000). In 25% of the cases, both chromosomes 15 originate from the mother (maternal uniparental disomy) and the regions q11-13 of these chromosomes are silenced (Nicolls et al. 1989). Speech is characterised by multiple articulation difficulties (consonant distortions associated with hypotonia and oral motor difficulties), voice difficulties (including impairment of frequency levels and resonance and hoarse voice quality), frequent hypernasality, slow speaking rate and markedly lowering speech intelligibility (Defloor et al. 2000). Dysfluencies are common but do not seem to conform completely to the pattern of stuttering. A mixed clinical picture emerges with features characteristic of stuttering (for example, within-word dysfluencies such as part-word repetitions, whole-word repetitions, blocks, prolongations, broken words; dysfluencies occurring more frequently on the first words of a sentence and being more prevalent in content than in function words) but none of the secondary symptoms of stuttering such as bodily movements (Defloor et al. 2000). Hearing problems are common. Receptive and expressive lexical and syntactic levels are found below CA expectations (Akefeldt et al. 1997). Language pragmatic skills and communicative efficiency are problematic (for example, excessive talkativeness and verbal perseverations on a narrow range of topics). Narrative retelling abilities are usually poor (Lewis et al. 2002).

ANGELMAN SYNDROME (AS)

This is another syndrome, like PWS, showing the effects of genomic imprinting. It has a prevalence of 1 in 20000 to 1 in 30000 births (Angelman 1965) or 1 in 12000 to 1 in 25000 (Kytterman 1995).

In 60% to 70% of the cases, AS is caused by the silencing of a number of genes in the q11-13 region of chromosome 15 of paternal origin (Christian et al. 1995) and the simultaneous deletion of the same genes on the maternal copy of the same chromosome (Lombroso 2000). In a small percentage of the cases (from 2% to 5%) the condition is the result of paternal uniparental disomy (inheritance of two copies of the above locus from the father and none from the mother; the pathology occurs when the whole region q11-13, or a part of it, is silenced). In 5% to 8% of the cases the molecular basis of the condition is found in mutations of one of the genes of the region q11-13 (UBE3A), which appears to be specifically expressed in the brain (Everman & Cassidy 2000). Level of intellectual disability varies from moderate to profound. Developmental delays are severe. Noticeable in AS is the absence or severe reduction of speech and oral language, together with oral dyspraxia (Penner et al. 1993), widely spaced teeth and protruding tongue. Nonverbal techniques of communication have been tried with limited success, suggesting that the capacity for language (not only speech) may be gravely impaired (Summers et al. 1995). Even at the prelinguistic level, major difficulties exist in joint attention, babbling, reciprocal interaction with caretakers, sound imitation, and imitation of mouth and lip movements (Brun Gasca et al. 2001). Andersen et al. (2002) report expressive verbal vocabulary consisting of less than two words in 50% of their cohort of AS (boys and girls aged 2 to 14 years), two to three words in 33% of the children, and four to five words in the remaining ones. Receptive abilities may be superior to expressive ones, at least in some cases (Thompson & Bolton 2003).

CRI-DU-CHAT SYNDROME (CDCS)

This is a rare syndrome (prevalence: approximately 1 case in 50000 newborns, not varying according to sex – Pueschel & Thuline 1991) caused by a loss of chromosomal material from the region 5p (Lejeune et al. 1963). Twenty per cent of the cases are familial, with parental translocation accounting for the majority of these. The rest of the cases occur spontaneously by a genetic mutation. Gersch et al. (1995) have determined that two distinct chromosomal regions are associated with differential phenotypic manifestations. Deletions in 5p15.3 result in the high-pitched cry characteristic of the syndrome. The typical facial dysmorphias are lacking and cognitive impairment is mild to moderate. In contrast, the loss of region 5p15.2, designated the cri-du-chat critical region (Overhauser et al. 1994) results in the full spectrum of CDCS.

The typical phenotype presents a characteristic monochromate cry at birth due to a laryngomalacia in most subjects but not persisting beyond 2 years in 30% of them; the rest of the subjects may present an acute and monochromatic tone of voice all their life. Other characteristics include dysmorphic craniofacial features with microcephaly, dental malocclusion, hypotonia, psychomotor retardation, slower rate of growth, respiratory and ear infections. People with CDCS demonstrate cognitive, language and motor deficits. Lack of speech may be observed in some cases. Limited verbal abilities and severe language problems are noted. However, many children with CDCS have the ability to develop at least some language but onset usually is markedly delayed (Sohner & Mitchell 1991). Cornish and Munir (1998) assessed the receptive and expressive abilities in a cohort of 14 CDCS individuals (males and females) aged 4 to 14 years. Except in one case, no subject's score on the British Picture Vocabulary Scales (Dunn et al. 1982) was CA appropriate. Three children failed to reach the 2-year baseline. All subjects were delayed in receptive grammar – some failed to reach the CA 4 years baseline – assessed with the Test of the Reception of Grammar (TROG) (Bishop 1983). Expressive language was markedly delayed (by several years) – equivalent scores on the Reynell Developmental Language Scales revised (Reynell 1985). At the time of testing, only one subject could speak in sentences of four or more words. A common pattern in CDCS is for receptive language skills to be better preserved than expressive ones across the various language components.

Other genetic syndromes of MR are more favourable to language, such as Turner syndrome or Klinefelter syndrome.

TURNER SYNDROME (TS)

This occurs in approximately 1 per 2500 births in females (Ross et al. 2000). About 60% of the females born with TS are missing one X chromosome (45X0 formula) whereas the remainder have a partial X chromosome or a mosaic chromosomal pattern (complete or partial monosomy). 47XXX cases also exist (Ginther & Fullwood 1998). All full, partial and mosaic 45X0 TS subjects lack ovarian oestrogen production as the result of the absence of defined gonads (Park et al. 1983). Mental retardation is uncommon but particular cognitive deficits are found in visuospatial processing (Ross et al. 1995). Oral language skills have often been described as preserved (Ross et al. 1995). However, Van Borsel et al. (1999) report frequent voice disorders, articulation problems, occasional stuttering, and overall delayed language development, in a sample of 128 girls with TS ranging in age from 2 years 4 months to 5 years 8 months. Murphy et al. (1994) found lower scores in tests of syntax comprehension in some TS individuals. Some TS females also have difficulty in tasks of verbal fluency (Money & Alexander 1986). Mosaic TS subjects, however, exhibit better cognitive and verbal abilities (Bender et al. 1984). Pennington et al. (1980) have indicated that 47XXX females do present with important language delays (longitudinal study conducted with unselected girls between birth and 14 years). Corresponding data regarding the existence of a significant deficit in verbal IQ in 47XXX children have been supplied by Netley & Rovet (1982).

KLINEFELTER SYNDROME (KS)

This is found exclusively in males presenting with one, two, or three extra X chromosomes (47XXY, 48XXXY, 49XXXXY), one extra Y chromosome (47XYY), or one extra X and one extra Y chromosome (48XXYY). The aneuploidies may be partial or complete and mosaicism may be involved. It affects one in 1000 births (Mandoki et al. 1991). The additional X chromosome is of paternal origin in 50% to 60% of the XXY births, with maternal origin occurring in the remaining cases. Klinefelter syndrome is characterised by a tall stature, decreased muscle tone, average intelligence, learning disability or mild MR (Walzer et al. 1991). Language problems are common, particularly on the expressive side. Verbal IQ tends to be depressed compared to nonverbal IQ (Netley & Rovet 1982). Delayed speech development during early childhood is frequent with prosodic difficulties. Word selection and sentence organisation are problematic in some cases (Leonard et al. 1979). The language difficulties are also a characteristic of adults with 47XXY, with scores significantly below controls in lexical abilities and verbal processing speed in a study of KS subjects aged 16 to 61 years by Brauer Boone et al. (2001). Severe retardation in language development (particularly regarding the expressive ability) in males with 49XXXXY has been reported by Moric-Petrovic et al. (1973) and confirmed by Curfs et al. (1990).

EXPLAINING SYNDROME SPECIFICITY

One reasonable possibility is that intersyndrome variability corresponds in major ways to differences in neurodevelopment and brain structures. Examination of DS brains reveals reductions in weight of the hemispheres, brain stem, and cerebellum, smaller overall brain and cerebellar volumes, relatively larger subcortical grey matter volumes, delays in myelinisation (primarily in the association cortex), reductions in number of neurons in the whole cerebral cortex and particularly in some cortical layers (Pinter et al. 2001). People with DS have reduced synaptic density and abnormal synaptic morphology and contacts (Wisniewski & Kida 1994). The presence of the above abnormalities from an early age in DS (cf. Pinter et al. 2001, using a higher resolution magnetic resonance imagery (MRI) study) suggests that foetal or early postnatal differences with normal neurogenesis underlie the observed patterns and abnormalities. The abnormal neurogenesis in DS may primarily reflect genetically determined altered brain programming.

Available studies point to important neurological differences between syndromes originating in different genetic bases. This may explain the specific fractionation of language functions observed in the phenotypes. Research suggests that functional differences between WS and DS individuals correspond to syndromic variation at brain level. Bellugi et al. (1990) compared the neurological profiles of WS and DS adolescents matched for CA and IQ. The WS subjects demonstrated generalised hypotonia, tremor, midline balance problems and motor abnormalities, suggestive of cerebellar dysfunction. Down syndrome adolescents showed minimal hypotonia, little evidence of palaeocerebellar signs, and better performance on oromotor functions. Both groups exhibited equal degrees of microcephaly, cerebral hypoplasia, reduced cerebral volume and decreased myelination but the overall brain shapes of each group proved distinct. Down syndrome brains exhibit important degrees of hypofrontality whereas WS individuals show relative preservation of anterior cortical areas but have decreased posterior width with reduction in size of the forebrain posterior to the rolandic sulcus – the posterior parietal, temporal (with relative preservation of mesial-temporal, however) and occipital cortical regions. Individuals with WS have elongated posterior to anterior length compared with normal brains, a greater ratio of frontal to posterior (parietal-occipital) tissue and disproportionate volume reduction of the brainstem (Reiss et al. 2000). Hypofrontality of neocortex in DS subjects, together with reduction in the frontal projections from the corpus callosum, was further demonstrated in a magnetic resonance imagery study by Wang et al. (1992). These authors relate this neuroanatomical indication to a profile of frontal lobe dysfunction in DS corresponding to poor verbal fluency, perseverative tendencies and greater difficulty on tasks requiring flexible problem-solving strategies. Individuals with DS, however, have relatively preserved basal ganglia and diencephalic structures (Bellugi et al.

2000). In contrast, WS subjects exhibit better frontal superior temporal gyrus volumes and temporal limbic structures (Jernigan et al. 1993). In WS, there is also evidence of dysregulation of the control of neuronal and glial numbers, as illustrated by increased cell packing density at the cytoarchitectonic level (Galaburda et al. 1994). This may reflect an interference with naturally occurring cell death and the presence of neurotrophic factors (possibly linked to abnormal extracellular calcium levels). A study by Schmitt et al. (2001a, b) throws further light on the anatomy of the corpus callosum in individuals with WS. Compared to CA-matched TD controls, WS subjects (aged between 19 and 44 years) showed significantly reduced total midsagittal corpus callosum. However, the splenium and isthmus areas were disproportionately reduced in WS beyond the absolute reduction of the entire corpus callosum (see also Tomaiulo et al. 2002). The reductions may be set in concordance with the decreased parieto-occipital volumes and functionally with the observed visuospatial problems existing in WS. Electrophysiological studies (for example, using the event-related potential sentence-processing technique) suggest abnormal patterns of cerebral specialisation for language treatment in persons with WS (Mills et al. 2000).

The cerebellar volume in DS subjects is approximately 77% of the equivalent in young normal controls versus 99% in WS subjects. Although cerebellar size is intact and the neocerebellum largely preserved or even enlarged in WS (Schmitt et al. 2001a, b), some other neurological findings suggest cerebellar dysfunction. The posterior fossa structures of the WS and DS subjects were further examined by Bellugi et al. (1990), leading to the identification, in WS, of an anomalous pattern with neocerebellar vermal lobules showing hyperplasia in the context of low-normal palaeocerebellar vermal development and significantly reduced forebrain size. Such an aberrant cerebrum/cerebellum volume ratio could serve to distinguish WS neurologically from other syndromes such as DS (Courchesne et al. 1988). Bellugi et al. (1990) speculate (in agreement with suggestions by Leiner et al. 1991, 1993 and Fabbro et al. 2000 regarding the possible role of human neocerebellar structures in linguistic functions) that the observed hyperplasia of specific verbal lobules in the context of cerebellar maldevelopment may be related to the language profile of WS subjects. Bellugi et al. (1990) further remark that their WS subjects were behaviourally similar to unilateral right-hemisphere damaged (normal) adults whereas the DS individuals were more like left-hemisphere damaged aphasics, demonstrating language impairment and a marked tendency towards more global information processing.

Neurological differences in other genetic syndromes have been studied less. Brain synaptic abnormalities have been documented (Wisniewski et al. 1991; Hinton et al. 1994) in many male subjects with FXS. Decreased posterior cerebellar vermis size has been observed (Hagerman 1996). As this neurological structure is involved with processing sensory stimuli and modulating motor activity, the indication is consistent with the motor deficits (Friefeld &

MacGregor 1993), as well as with the inattention, hyperactivity, and hypersensitivity to stimuli, seen in many FXS males (Mostofsky et al. 1998). Decreased amounts of FMRP (the FMR-1 protein) impair the development of the cerebellum Purkinje cells, the cholinergic neurons innervating the limbic system (involved in emotional and mood regulation) and other neuronal tissues (grey matter particularly) that normally exhibit high concentrations of FMRP. Conversely, in males and females with FXS, there are enlargements of some brain structures such as the hippocampus (a major convergence zone in the cortex involved, among other things, in the storage and consolidation of long-term declarative memories) the ventricles, the thalamus, and the caudate nucleus (Reiss et al. 1995). These findings may be associated with impulsivity perseverations, stereotypies, hyperactivity, attentional impairment and other problems in planning and executive functions such as inhibiting responses, regulating affect and motor activity, whose speech and language effects are typically observed (Abrams & Reiss 1995; Hatton et al. 1999). Head circumference is typically large in male FXS individuals, in contrast to the microcephaly found in DS and many other MR syndromes. There is enlargement of some brain structures (for example, the hippocampus), probably linked to a defect in synaptic priming early in brain development (Rakic et al. 1994; Hagerman 1996). Another and possibly complementary hypothesis suggests that abnormalities in the frontal lobe result in a difficulty inhibiting high strength, salient, or previously activated responses (Abbeduto & Hagerman 1997).

In RS, electrophysiology demonstrates progressively abnormal electroencephalograms. Neurometabolic factors including reduced levels of dopamine, serotonin, noradrenaline and choline acetyltransferase in the brain have been documented (Dunn 2001). Hyperfunction of the aminergic neurons (noradrenaline, serotonin, and dopamine in the brainstem and midbrain) has been suggested as the main cause of dysfunction of the neuronal systems involving primarily locomotion and hand use, and secondarily the development of language and cognitive functions (Segawa 2001).

Regarding KS, Geschwind et al. (2000) propose that altered left-hemisphere functioning, whether causing or due to altered functional and anatomical cerebral dominance, is at the core of KS individuals' language problems. The observations regarding individuals with KS suggest that one major contributory factor may be the X or Y chromosome because in the polysomy disorders of KS there is only one active X or Y and the additional X, Xs or Y undergo inactivation to some extent (Willard 1995), whereas a number of genes on the active chromosomes X and Y are altered by the existence of the polysomy (Geschwind et al. 2000).

A neurogenetic perspective can explain the differences between XO (TS) and other sex chromosome anomaly disorders as well as the basic similarities among disorders such as XXY, XXXY, XXXXY, XYY and XXYY. The variability in individuals with KS may also be related to the impact of gonadal steroids. Patwardhan et al. (2000) have measured regional brain volumes with high-resolution MRI in a cohort of 10 young adults with 47XXY KS and 10 CA controls. They document a significantly lower volume in left temporal grey matter volumes in KS subjects when compared with normal control subjects. Differences in left temporal grey matter volume were also significant between the KS subjects treated with exogenous testosterone supplementation since puberty and those KS subjects who did not receive this treatment.

For TS, Murphy et al. (1997) suggest that the generalised brain hypermetabolism they observed in young female adults reflects global abnormalities in neuron packing whereas the lower regional metabolism observed in the association cortices reflects neuronal abnormalities related to the cognitive deficits typical of the condition.

CONCLUSION

The preceding analyses, which are still preliminary in many respects, encourage the belief that considerable insight into the genetic syndromes of MR and some of the mechanisms responsible for language development, its difficulties and defects, can be gained from a perspective oriented towards specifying the neurobehavioural particulars as well as the similarities of the various syndromes. Individuals with DS, as well as other syndromes of genetic origin, typically present enough distinctive speech and language features to justify a specific approach regarding interventions. It is likely that these particulars are in close relation with (and are largely caused by) distinctive brain features originating in the genotypes. The more we know about these features the better able we will be to design more efficient therapies.

REFERENCES

Abbeduto, L., Hagerman, R. (1997) Language and communication in fragile X syndrome. *Ment Retard Dev Disabil*, **3**, 313–322.

Abrams, M., Reiss, A. (1995) The neurobiology of fragile X syndrome. *Ment Retard Dev Disabil*, **1**, 269–275.

Akefeldt, A., Akefeldt, B., Gillberg, C. (1997) Voice, speech, and language characteristics of children with Prader-Willi syndrome. *J Intellect Disabil Res*, **41**, 302–311.

Andersen, W., Rasmussen, R., Stromme, P. (2002) Levels of cognitive and linguistic development in Angelman syndrome: a study of 20 children. *Logopedics and Phonology*, **26**, 2–9.

Angelman, H. (1965) 'Puppet' children: a report on three cases. *Dev Med Child Neurol*, **7**, 681–688.

Auranen, M., Vanhala, R., Vosman, M., Levander, M., Varilo, T., Hietala, M., et al. (2001) MECP2 gene analysis in classical Rett syndrome and in patients with Rett-like features. *Neurology*, **56**, 611–617.

Bailey, D., Hatton, D. Tassone, F., Skinner, M., Taylor, A. (2001) Variability in FMRP and early development in males with Fragile X syndrome. *Am J Mental Retard*, **106**, 16–27.

Bellugi, U., Bihrle, A., Jernigan, T., Trauner, D., Doherty, S. (1990) Neuropsychological, neurological and neuro-anatomical profile of Williams syndrome. *Am J Med Genet Suppl*, **6**, 115–125.

Bellugi, U., Lichtenberger, L., Jones, W., Lai, Z., St George, M. (2000) The neuro-cognitive profile of Williams syndrome: a complex pattern of strengths and weaknesses. *J Cognit Neurosci*, **12**, 7–29.

Bellugi, U., Marks, S., Bihrle, A., Sabo, H. (1988) Dissociation between language and cognitive functions in Williams syndrome. In D. Bishop, K. Mogford (eds) *Language Development in Exceptional Circumstances*. London: Churchill Livingstone, pp. 177–189.

Bender, B., Puck, M., Salbenblatt, J., Robinson, A. (1984) Cognitive development of unselected girls with complete and partial monosomy. *Pediatrics*, **73**, 175–182.

Bishop, D. (1983) *Test of the Reception of Grammar*. London: Medical Research Council.

Borgraef, M., Fryns, J.-P., Dielkens, A., Pyck, K., Van den Berghe, H. (1987) Fragile-X syndrome: a study of psychological profile in 23 prepubertal patients. *Clin Genet*, **32**, 179–186.

Boudreau, D., Chapman, R. (2000) The relationship between event representation and linguistic skill in narratives of children and adolescents with Down syndrome. *Journal of Speech, Language, and Hearing Research*, **43**, 1146–1159.

Brauer Boone, K., Swerdloff, R., Miller, B., Geschwind, D., Razani, J., Lee, A., et al. (2001) Neuropsychological profiles of adults with Klinefelter syndrome. *J Int Neuropsychol Soc*, **7**, 446–456.

Brun Gasca, C., Conesa Perez, M., Torres Gil, M. (2001) Retraso mental de base genetica: caracteristicas de lenguaje. *Revista de Logopedia, Foniatria y Audiologia*, **21**, 81–85.

Butler, M., Meaney, F., Palmer, C. (1986) Clinical and cytogenetic survey of 39 individuals with Prader-Willi syndrome. *Am J Med Genet*, **23**, 793–809.

Capirci, O., Sabbadini, L., Volterra, V. (1996) Language development in Williams syndrome: a case study. *Cognitive Neuropsychology*, **13**, 1017–1039.

Capone, G. (2001) Down syndrome: advances in molecular biology and the neuro-sciences. *Dev Behav Pediatr*, **22**, 40–59.

Cardoso-Martins, C., Mervis, C. B., Mervis, C. A. (1985) Early vocabulary acquisition by children with Down's syndrome. *Am J Ment Defic*, **89**, 451–458.

Cassidy, S. (1997) Prader-Willi syndrome. *Journal of Medical Genetics*, **34**, 917–923.

Chapman, R., Schwartz, S., Kay-Raining Bird, E. (1991) Fast-mapping in stories: Deficits in Down's syndrome. Communication at the Annual Meeting of the American Speech-Language-Hearing Association, Atlanta GA, November 1991.

Christian, S., Robinson, W., Huang, B., Mutirangrera, A., Liuc, M., Nakao, M., et al. (1995) Molecular characterization of two proximal deletion breakpoint regions in both Prader-Willi and Angelman syndrome patients. *Am J Hum Genet*, **57**, 40–48.

Coggins, T., Carpenter, R., Owings, N. (1983) Examing early intentional communication in Down's syndrome and nonretarded children. *British Journal of Disorders of Communication*, **18**, 99–107.

Cornish, K., Munir, F. (1998) Receptive and expressive language skills in children with cri-du-chat syndrome. *J Comm Disord*, **31**, 73–81.

Courchesne, E., Yeung-Courchesne, R., Press, G., Hesselink, J., Jernigan, T. (1988) Hypophasia of cerebellar vermal lobules VI and II in autism. *New Engl J Med*, **318**, 1349–1354.

Curfs, L., Schreppers-Tijdink, G., Wiegers, A., Borghraef, M., Fryns, J. P. (1990) The 49,XXXXY syndrome: clinical and psychologocial findings in five patients. *J Ment Defic Res*, **34**, 277–282.

Daniel, L., Gridley, B. (1998) Prader-Willi syndrome. In L. Phelps (ed.) *A Guidebook for Understanding and Educating Health-related Disorders in Children and Adolescents. A Compilation of 96 Rare and Common Disorders.* Washington DC: American Psychological Association, pp. 534–540.

Defloor, T., Van Borsel, J., Curfs, L. (2000) Speech fluency in Prader-Willi syndrome. *Journal of Fluency Disorders*, **25**, 85–98.

Dodd, B., Leahy, J. (1989) Phonological disorders and mental handicap. In M. Beveridge, G. Conti-Ramsden, Y. Leudar (eds) *Language and Communication in Mentally Handicapped People.* London: Chapman & Hall, pp. 35–56.

Dunn, H. (2001) Importance of Rett syndrome in child neurology. *Brain and Development*, 23, S38–S43.

Dunn, L., Dunn, P., Whetton, C., Pintilie, D. (1982) *British Picture Vocabulary Scales.* Windsor: NFER-Nelson.

Dykens, E., Cassidy, S. (1996) Prader-Willi syndrome: genetic, behavioral, and treatment issues. *Child and Adolescent Psychiatric Clinics of North America*, **5**, 913–927.

Dykens, E., Hodapp, R., Finucane, B. (2000) *Genetics and Mental Retardation Syndromes.* Baltimore: Brookes.

Everman, D., Cassidy, S. (2000) Genetics of childhood disorders: XII. Genomic imprinting: breaking the rules. *Journal of the American Academy of Child and Adolescent Psychiatry*, **39**, 386–389.

Fabbro, F., Moretti, R., Bava, A. (2000) Language impairments in patients with cerebellar lesions. *Journal of Neurolinguistics*, **13**, 173–188.

Fishler, K., Koch, R. (1991) Mental development in Down syndrome mosaicism. *Am J Ment Retard*, **96**, 345–351.

Friefeld, S., MacGregor, D. (1993) Sensory-motor coordination in boys with fragile X syndrome. In J. A. Holden, B. Cameron (eds) *Proceeedings of the First Canadian Fragile X Conference.* Kingston, Ontario: Oudwanda Resource Center, pp. 59–65.

Galaburda, A., Wang, P., Bellugi, U., Rosen, M. (1994) Cytoarchitectonic anomalies in a genetically based disorder: Williams syndrome. *Cognitive Neuroscience and Neuropsychology*, **5**, 753–757.

Gerard, C. L., Guillotte, E., Servel, E., Barbeau, M. (1997) Evaluation et rééducation des troubles de la communication chez les enfants porteurs d'un syndrome de l'X fragile. *Approches Neuropsychologiques des Apprentissages de l'Enfant*, **45**, 224–226.

Gersch, M., Goodhart, S., Paszter, L., Harris, D., Weiss, L., Overhauser, J. (1995) Evidence for a distinct region causing a cat-like cry in patients with 5p deletions. *Am J Hum Genet*, **56**, 1404–1410.

Geschwind, D., Boone, K., Miller, B., Swerdloft, R. (2000) Neurobehavioral phenotype of Klinefelter syndrome. *Mental Retardation and Developmental Disability Research Review*, **6**, 107–116.

Ginther, D., Fullwood, H. (1998) Turner's syndrome. In L. Phelps (ed.) *A Guidebook for Understanding and Educating Health-related Disorders in Children and Adolescents. A Compilation of 96 Rare and Common Disorders.* Washington DC: American Psychological Association, pp. 691–695.

Greenwald, C., Leonard, L. (1979) Communicative and sensorimotor development of Down's syndrome children. *Am J Ment Defic*, **84**, 296–303.

Hagerman, R. (1996) Biomedical advances in developmental psychology: the case of fragile X syndrome. *Dev Psychol*, **32**, 416–424.

Hatton, D., Bailey, D., Hargett-Beck, M., Skinner, M., Clark, R. (1999) Behavioral style of young boys with fragile X syndrome. *Dev Med Child Neurol*, **41**, 625–632.

Hinton, V., Brown, T., Wisniewski, K., Rudelli, D. (1994) Analysis of neocortex in three males with the fragile X syndrome. *Am J Med Genet*, **41**, 289–294.

Hodapp, R., Dykens, E., Finucane, B. (2000) *Genetics and Mental Retardation.* Baltimore MD: Brookes.

Jernigan, T., Bellugi, U., Sowell, E., Doherty, S., Hesselink, J. (1993) Cerebral morphologic distinctions between Williams and Down's syndromes. *Arch Neurol*, **50**, 186–191.

Kerr, A., Corbitt, J. (1994) Rett syndrome: from gene to gesture. *J Roy Soc Med*, **87**, 562–566.

Korenberg, J., Chen, X., Hirota, H., Lai, Z., Bellugi, U., Burian, D., et al. (2000) Genome structure and cognitive map of Williams syndrome. *J Cognit Neurosci*, **12**, 89–107.

Kumin, L. (2001) Speech intelligibility in individuals wi!th Down syndrome: a framework for targeting specific factors for assessment and treatment. *Down Syndrome Quarterly*, **6**, 1–8.

Kytterman, M. (1995) On the prevalence of Angelman syndrome. *Am J Med Genet*, **59**, 405.

Leiner, C., Leiner, A., Dow, R. (1991) The human cerebro-cerebellar system: its computing, cognitive, and language skills. *Behav Brain Res*, **44**, 113–128.

Leiner, C., Leiner, A., Dow, R. (1993) Cognitive and language functions of the human cerebellum. *Trends Neurosci*, **16**, 444–447.

Lejeune, J., Lafourcade, J., Berger, R. (1963) Trois cas de délétion partielle du bras court d'un chromosome 5. *Compte Rendus de l'Académie des Science de Paris*, **257**, 3098–3102.

Leonard, M., Schowalter, J. E., Landy, G., Ruddle, F. H., Lubs, H. A. (1979) Chromosomal abnormalities in the New Haven newborn study: a prospective study of development of children with sex chromosome anomalies. In A. Robinson, H. A. Lubs, D. Bergsma (eds) *Birth Defects.* New York: Alan R. Liss, pp. 115–159.

Lewis, B., Freebairn, L., Heeger, S., Cassidy, S. (2002) Speech and language skills of individuals with Prader-Willi syndrome. *Am J Speech Lang*, **11**, 285–294.

Lombroso, P. (2000) Genetics of childhood disorders: XVI. Angelman syndrome: a failure to process. *Journal of the American Academy of Child and Adolescent Psychiatry*, **39**, 931–933.

Maes, B., Fryns, J. P., Van Walleghem, M., Van den Berghe, H. (1994) Cognitive functioning and information processing of adult mentally retarded with fragile X syndrome. *Am J Med Genet*, **50**, 190–200.

Mandoki, M., Summer, G., Hoffman, R., Riconda, D. (1991) A review of Klinefelter's syndrome in children and adolescents. *Journal of American Academy of Child and Adolescent Psychiatry*, **30**, 167–172.

Markman, E. (1990) Constraints children place on word meanings. *Cognit Sci*, **14**, 57–77.

Martin, N., Snodgrass, G., Cohen, R. (1984) Idiopathic infantile hypercalcaemia – a continuing enigma. *Archives of Diseases in Childhood*, **59**, 605–613.

Mervis, C., Robinson, B. (2005) Designing measures for profiling and genotype phenotype studies of individuals with genetic syndromes or developmental language disorders. *Applied Psycholinguistics*, **26**, 41–64.

Mervis, C., Robinson, B., Rowe, M., Becerra, A., Klein-Tasman, B. (2003) Language ability of individuals with Williams syndrome. In L. Abbeduto (ed.) Language and communication in mental retardation. *International Review of Research in Mental Retardation*, Vol. 28. New York: Academic, pp. 35–81.

Miles, S., Chapman, R. (2002) Narrative content as described by individuals with Down syndrome and typically developing children. *Journal of Speech, Language, and Hearing Research*, **45**, 175–189.

Miller, J. (1999) Profiles of language development in children with Down syndrome. In J. Miller, M., Leddy, L. Leavitt (eds) *Improving the Communication of People with Down Syndrome*. Baltimore MD: Brookes, pp. 11–39.

Mills, D., Alvarez, T., St George, M., Appelbaum, L., Bellugi, U., Neville, H. (2000) Electrophysiological studies of face processing in Williams syndrome. *J Cognit Neurosci*, **12** supplement: 47–64.

Money, J., Alexander, D. (1986) Turner's syndrome: Further demonstration of the presence of specific cognitional deficiencies. *J Med Genet*, **3**, 47–48.

Moric-Petrovic, S., Laca, Z., Markovic, S., Markovic, V. (1973) 49, XXXXY karyotype in a mentally retarded boy. *J Ment Def Res*, **17**, 73–80.

Mostofsky, S., Mazzocco, M., Aakalu, G., Warsofsky, I., Denkla, M., Reiss, A. (1998) Decreased cerebellar posterior vermis size in Fragile X syndrome: correlation with neurocognitive performance. *Neurology*, **50**, 121–130.

Murphy, D., Allen, G., Haxby, J., Largay, K., Daly, E., White, B., et al. (1994) The effects of sex steroids and the X chromosome on female brain function: a study of the neuropsycology of adult Turner syndrome. *Neuropsychologia*, **32**, 1309–1323.

Murphy, D., Mentis, M., Pietrini, P., Grady, C., Daly, E., Haxby, J., et al. (1997) A PET study of Turner's syndrome: effects of sex steroids and the X chromosome on brain. *Biol Psychiatr* **41**, 285–298.

Murphy, M., Abbeduto, L. (2003) Language and communication in Fragile X syndrome. In L. Abbeduto (ed.) Language and communication in mental retardation. *International Review of Research in Mental Retardation*, Vol. 27, New York: Academic, pp. 83–119.

Nazzi, T., Karmiloff-Smith, A. (2002) Early categorization abilities in young children with Williams syndrome. *Cognitive Neuroscience and Neuropsychology*, **13**, 1259–1262.

Nazzi, T., Paterson, S., Karmiloff-Smith, A. (2003) Early word segmentation by infants and toddlers with Williams syndrome. *Infancy*, **4**, 251–271.

Netley, C., Rovet, J. (1982) Verbal deficits in children with 47,XXY and 47,XXX karyotypes: a descriptive and experimental study. *Brain Lang*, **17**, 58–72.

Nicholls, R., Knoll, J., Buther, M. Karam, S., Lalander, M. (1989) Genetic imprinting suggested by maternal heterodisomy in nondeletion Prader-Willi syndrome. *Nature*, **342**, 281–285.

O'Neill, M., Henry, A. (2002) The grammatical morpheme difficulty in Down's syndrome. *Belfast Working Papers in Language and Linguistics*, **15**, 65–72.

Overhauser, J., Huang, X., Gersch, M., Wilson, W., McMahon, J., Bengtsson, U., et al. (1994) Molecular and phenotypic mapping of the short arm of chromosome 5: sublocalization of the critical region for the cri-du-chat syndrome. *Hum Mol Genet*, **34**, 247–252.

Owens, R., MacDonald, J. (1982) Communicative uses of the early speech of nondelayed and Down syndrome children. *Am J Ment Defic*, **86**, 503–510.

Park, E., Bailey, J., Cowell, C. (1983) Growth and maturation of patients with Turner syndrome. *Pediatr Res*, **17**, 1–7.

Patwardhan, A., Eliez, S., Bender, B., Linden, M., Reiss, A. (2000) Brain morphology in Klinefelter syndrome. *Neurology*, **54**, 2218–2223.

Penner, K., Johnston, J., Faircloth, B., Irish, P., Williams, C. (1993) Communication, cognition, and social interaction in Angelman syndrome. *Am J Med Genet*, **46**, 34–39.

Pennington, B. (1995) Genetics of learning disabilities. *J Child Neurol*, **10**, S69–S78.

Pennington, B., Puck, M., Robinson, A. (1980) Language and cognitive development in 47, XXX females followed since birth. *Behav Genet*, **10**, 31–41.

Pinter, J., Eliez, S., Schmitt, J., Capone, G., Reiss, A. (2001) Neuroanatomy of Down's syndrome, a high-resolution MRI study. *Am J Psychiatr*, **158**, 1659–1665.

Pueschel, S., Thuline, H. (1991) Chromosome disorders. In J. Matson, J. Mulick (eds) *Handbook of Mental Retardation*. Elmsford NY: Pergamon, pp. 115–138.

Rakic, P., Bourgeois, J.-P., Goldman-Rakic, P. S. (1994) Synaptic development of the cerebral cortex: implications for learning, memory, and metal illness. *Prog Brain Res*, **102**, 227–243 (special issue).

Reilly, J., Klima, E., Bellugi, U. (1990) Once more with feeling: affect and language in atypical populations. *Developmental Psychopathology*, **2**, 367–391.

Reiss, A., Abrams, M., Greenlaw, R., Freund, L., Denkla, M. (1995) Neurodevelopmental effects of the FMR-1 full mutations in humans. *Nat Med*, **1**, 159–167.

Reiss, A., Eliez, J., Schmitt, E., Straus, E., Lai, Z., Jones, W., et al. (2000) Neuroanatomy of Williams syndrome: a high-resolution MR1 study. *J Cognit Neurosci*, **12**, 65–73.

Reynell, J. (1985) *Reynell Developmental Language Scales*. Windsor, UK: NFER-Nelson.

Roberts, J., Mirrett, P., Burchinal, M. (2001) Receptive and expressive communicatin development of young males with Fragile X syndrome. *Am J Ment Retard*, **106**, 216–230.

Rondal, J. A. (1978) Maternal speech to normal and Down's syndrome children matched for mean length of utterance. In C. Meyers (ed.) *Quality of Life in the Severely and Profoundly Retarded People: Research Foundations for Improvement*. Washington DC: American Association on Mental Deficiency, pp. 193–265.

Rondal, J. A. (1995) *Exceptional Language Development in Down Syndrome: Implications for the Cognition-language Relationship*. Cambridge MA: Cambridge University Press.

Rondal, J. A. (2003) Atypical language development in individuals with mental retardation: theoretical implications. In L. Abbeduto (ed.) Language and communication. *International Review of Research in Mental Retardation*, Vol. 27. New York: Academic, pp. 281–308.

Rondal, J. A. (2004) Intersyndrome and intrasyndrome language differences. In J. A. Rondal, R. Hodapp, S. Soresi, E. Dykens, L. Nota, *Intellectual Disabilities. Genetics, Behaviour and Inclusion*. London: Whurr, pp. 49–113.

Rondal, J. A., Comblain, A. (1996) Language in adults with Down syndrome. *Down Syndrome*, **4**, 3–14.

Rondal, J. A., Comblain, A. (in press) Approche neuropsychologique des syndromes développementaux associés au chromosome X. In M. Poncelet, S. Majerus, M. van der Linden (eds) *Traité de neuropsychologie de l'enfant*. Marseille: Solal.

Rondal, J. A., Edwards, S. (1997) *Language in Mental Retardation*. London: Whurr.

Rondal, J. A., Hodapp, R., Soresi, S., Dykens, S., Nota, L. (2004) *Intellectual Disabilities: Genetics, Behaviour and Inclusion*. London: Whurr.

Rosenberg, S., Abbeduto, L. (1993) *Language and Communication in Mental Retardation. Development, Processes, and Intervention*. Hillsdale NJ: Erlbaum.

Ross, J., Roeltgen, D., Feuillan, P., Kushner, H., Cutler, G. (2000) Use of estrogen in young girls with Turner syndrome. *Neurology*, **54**, 164–170.

Ross, J., Stefanatos, G., Roeltgen, D., Kushner, H., Cutler, G. (1995) Ulrich-Turner syndrome: neurodevelopmental charges from childhood through adolescence. *Am J Med Genet*, **58**, 74–82.

Schmitt, J., Eliez, S., Warsofsky, I., Bellugi, U., Reiss, A. (2001a) Enlarged cerebellar vermis in Williams syndrome. *J Psychiatr Res*, **35**, 225–229.

Schmitt, J., Eliez, S., Warsofsky, I., Bellugi, U., Reiss, A. (2001b) Corpus callosum morphology of Williams syndrome: relation to genetics and behavior. *Dev Med Child Neurol*, **43**, 155–159.

Segawa, M. (2001) Pathophysiology of Rett syndrome from the stand point of clinical characteristics. *Brain and Development*, **23**, S94–S98.

Shprintzen, R. (1997) *Genetics Syndrome and Communication Disorders*. San Diego CA: Singular.

Smith, B. L., Oller, K. (1981) A comparative study of pre-meaningful vocalizations produced by normally developing and Down's syndrome infants. *Journal of Speech and Hearing Disorders*, **46**, 46–51.

Sohner, L., Mitchell, P. (1991) Phonatory and phonetic characteristics of prelinguistic vocal development in cri du chat syndrome. *J Comm Disord*, **24**, 10–13.

Spinelli, M., Oliveira Rocha, A., Giacheti, C., Richieri-Costa, A. (1995) Word-finding difficulties, verbal paraphasias, and verbal dyspraxia in ten individuals with fragile X syndrome. *Am J Med Genet*, **60**, 39–43.

Stevens, T., Karmiloff-Smith, A. (1997) Word learning in special population: do individuals with Williams syndrome obey lexical constraints? *J Child Lang*, **24**, 737–765.

Stiles, J., Sabbadini, L., Capirci, D., Volterra, V. (2000) Drawing abilities in Williams syndrome: a case study. *Dev Neuropsychol*, **18**, 213–235.

Sudhalter, V., Scarborough, H., Cohen, I. (1991) Syntactic delay and pragmatic deviance in the language of males with fragile X syndrome. *Am J Med Genet*, **43**, 65–71.

Summers, J., Allison, D., Lynch, P., Sandler, L. (1995) Behaviour problems in Angelman syndrome. *J Intellect Disabil Res*, **39**, 97–106.

Thomas, M., Grant, J., Barham, Z., Gsödl, M., Laing, E., Lakusta, L., et al. (2001) Past tense formation in Williams syndrome. *Language and Cognitive Processes*, **16**, 143–176.

Thompson, R., Bolton, P. (2003) Case report: Angelman syndrome in an individual with a s SMC15 and paternal uniparental disomy. A case report with reference to the assessment of cognitive functioning and autistic symptomatology. *J Autism Dev Disord*, **33**, 171–176.

Tomaiulo, F., Di Paola, M., Caravale, B., Vicari, S., Petrides, M., Caltagirone, C. (2002) Morphology and morphometry of the corpus callosum in Williams syndrome: ATI-weighted MRI study. *Clin Neurosci*, **13**, 2281–2284.

Trevathan, E., Moser, H. (1988) Diagnostic criteria for Rett syndrome. *Ann Neurol*, **23**, 425–428.

Turner, G., Webb, T., Wake, S., Robinson, H. (1996) Prevalence of the fragile X syndrome. *Am J Med Genet*, **64**, 196–197.

Van Borsel, J., Dhooge, I., Verhoye, K., Derde, K., Curfs, L. (1999) Communication problems in Turner syndrome: a sample survey. *J Comm Disord*, **32**, 435–446.

Van Borsel, J., Dor, O., Rondal, J. A. (2005) Fluency disorders in Fragile X syndrome. Communication presented at the Annual Conference of the American Speech and Hearing Association, San Diego CA, November 2005.

Verkerk, A., Pieretti, M., Sutcliffe, J., Fu, Y., Kuhi, D., Pizzuti, A., et al. (1991) Identification of a gene (FMR-1) containing a CHGG repeat coincident with a breakpoint cluster region exhibiting right variation in fragile X syndrome. *Cell*, **65**, 905–914.

Vilkman, E., Niemi, J., Ikonen, U. (1988) Fragile-X speech in Finnish. *Brain and Language*, **34**, 203–221.

Volterra, V., Capirci, O., Pezzini, G., Sabbadini, L., Vicari, S. (1994) Linguistic abilities in Italian children with Williams syndrome. Paper presented at the Sixth International Professional Conference, San Diego CA, July 1994.

Volterra, V., Caselli, C., Capirci, O., Tonucci, F., Vicari, S. (2003) Early linguistic abilities of Italian children with Williams syndrome. *Dev Neuropsychol*, **23**, 33–58.

Waltzer, S., Bashir, A., Silber, A. (1991) Cognitive and behavioral factors in the learning disabilites of 47XXY and 47XYY boys. *Birth Defects*, **26**, 45–58.

Wang, P., Doherty, S., Hesselink, J., Bellugi, U. (1992) Callosal morphology concurs with neuropathological findings in two neurodevelopmental disorders. *Arch Neurol*, **49**, 407–411.

Webb, T., Bundey, S., Thake, A., Todd, J. (1986) Population incidence and segregation ratios in Martin-Bell syndrome. *Am J Med Genet*, **23**, 573–580.

Willard, H. (1995) The sex chromosomes and X chromosome inactivation. In C. Schiver, A. Beaudet, W. Sly, D. Valli (eds) *The Metabolic and Molecular Basis of Inherited Disease*. New York: McGraw Hill, pp. 719–735.

Wishart, J. (1988) Early learning in infants and young children with Down syndrome. In L. Nadel (ed.) The Psychobiology of Down Syndrome. Cambridge MA: MIT Press, pp. 7–50.

Wisniewski, K., Kida, E. (1994) Abnormal neurogenesis and synaptogenesis in Down syndrome brain. *Dev Brain Dysfunct*, **17**, 1–12.

Wisniewski, K., Segan, S., Miezejeski, C., Searson, E., Rudelli, R. (1991) The Fra(X) syndrome: neurological, electrophysiological, and neuropathological abnormalities. *Am J Med Genet*, **38**, 476–480.

Witt-Engerstrom, I. (1987) Rett syndrome: a retrospective pilot study on potential early predictive symptomatology. *Brain and Development*, **9**, 481–486.

Wolf-Schein, E., Sudhalter, V., Cohen, I., Fisch, G., Hanson, D., Pfadt, A., et al. (1987) Speech-language and the fragile X syndrome. *Journal of the American Speech-Language-Hearing Association*, **29**, 35–38.

Xiang, F., Buervenich, S., Nicolao, P., Bailey, M., Zhang, Z., Anvret, M. (2000) Mutation screening in Rett syndrome patients. *J Med Genet*, **37**, 250–255.

Yamashita, Y., Kondo, I., Fukuda, T., Morishima, R., Kusaga, A., Iwanaga, R., et al. (2001) Mutation analysis of the methyl-CpG-binding protein 2 gene (MECP2) in Rett patients with preserved speech. *Brain and Development*, **23**, S157–S160.

Zappella, M. (1997) The preserved speech variant of the Rett complex: a report of 8 cases. *Eur J Child Adolesc Psychiatr*, **6**, 23–25.

8 Total versus Partial Specificity in the Behaviour of Persons with Down Syndrome

ROBERT M. HODAPP

Vanderbilt University, Nashville, USA

SUMMARY

In different syndromes involving intellectual disabilities (IDs), total specificity can be seen in individual behaviours, in profiles of relative strengths and weaknesses and in changing trajectories or rates of development. Although few unique individual behaviours seem evident in Down syndrome (DS), most people with the syndrome do show specific profiles of abilities: difficulties in language (especially in expressive language and grammar); better visual short-term memory than auditory short-term memory, and difficulties in long-term memory for episodic events. The syndrome also seems noteworthy for its 'fragile' development and for its sociability, which is often used to avoid performing difficult problems. In future years we need more studies on the issues of uniqueness and total specificity, development of the syndrome's behavioural phenotype and associations between aetiology-related profiles/trajectories and underlying brain functioning and interventions for children with DS.

INTRODUCTION

Since the mid-1980s, increased attention has been paid to behaviour in different genetic syndromes with IDs. In certain syndromes – for example, Prader-Willi syndrome, Williams syndrome, and fragile-X syndrome – the amount of research attention has increased exponentially from the 1980s to 1990s and into the new century. Even in DS, a disorder that has been studied for over 100 years (Gibson 1978), there have recently been increased numbers of behavioural studies. In a PsychLit search, Hodapp and Dykens (2004) noted that the numbers of behavioural research articles in DS increased from

Down Syndrome: Neurobehavioural Specificity. Edited by JA Rondal and J Perera.
© 2006 John Wiley & Sons Ltd.

607 to 1140 from the 1980s to the 1990s. The age of aetiology-based behavioural studies is upon us.

As explored throughout this volume, a key question in these studies relates to the uniqueness or 'total specificity' of any aetiology-based findings (Hodapp 1997). Simply stated, are the specific behavioural characteristics found in such studies unique to a single syndrome? Conversely, might such behaviours show themselves in other genetic disorders, or among all children with intellectual disabilities? Even if certain behavioural characteristics are unique to a single syndrome, how can we make use of such aetiology-related behaviours to understand gene-brain-behaviour relations or to intervene more effectively?

This chapter examines these issues vis-à-vis DS. I begin by discussing general issues involving the search for unique, totally specific behaviours in different genetic syndromes. Down syndrome is then examined more specifically before I explore several remaining issues.

TOTAL SPECIFICITY: SOME GENERAL ISSUES

To discuss the issue of total specificity more generally, it is first necessary to provide definitions, guidelines, and examples of behavioural characteristics.

DEFINITION

By definition, a totally specific connection between a genetic disorder and a behavioural outcome involves a unique connection, a connection found in no other genetic intellectual disability condition. We are here discussing so-called one-to-one connections, such that a single genetic disorder predisposes individuals with that disorder to show a specific, unique behavioural characteristic. Pennington et al. (1991) referred to this issue as the 'uniqueness question' (see also Wagner et al. 1990).

It is also noteworthy that the uniqueness prediction resembles the fairly restrictive definition of behavioural phenotypes first promulgated by Flint & Yule (1994). According to these workers, 'a behavioural phenotype should consist of a distinct behaviour that occurs in almost every case of a genetic or chromosomal disorder, and rarely (if at all) in other conditions' (Flint & Yule 1994, p. 666). Again, a one-to-one connection is being proposed: a link between a single genetic disorder and a specific behavioural outcome.

LOGICAL IMPOSSIBILITY OF MANY UNIQUE OUTCOMES

Given this definition of total specificity, it is important to state the obvious: it is logically impossible to have unique, totally specific outcomes for all syndromes in all aspects of behaviour. There are too few behavioural out-comes and too many genetic causes of intellectual disability.

Consider, first, the number of behavioural outcomes in almost any subarea of behaviour. Within intelligence, for example, there is likely a large 'general' factor (historically referred to as the 'g' factor in intelligence) as well as smaller subareas ('s' or specific factors) relating to such things as verbal versus performance or sequential versus simultaneous processing (Anderson 2001). Within maladaptive behaviour, Achenbach (1991) identifies external-ising and internalising behaviours as his two 'wide-band factors', with nine 'narrow-band' factors focusing on more specific areas of difficulty. Within personality, Costa & McRae (1992, 1997) have identified 'the big five' per-sonality factors of neuroticism, extraversion, openness to experience, agree-ableness, and conscientiousness. These factors have been found repeatedly in studies of individuals of different ages and with different emotional-behavioural problems.

In essence, individuals can vary on any domain of human behaviour in only a finite number of ways. Looking at profiles of strengths and weaknesses in verbal versus nonverbal intelligence, for example, one can be high on verbal and low on nonverbal intelligence; high on nonverbal and low on verbal; or close to the same on both domains. In the same way, there are small numbers of discrete profiles whenever an area of behaviour has only a few separate subdomains or factors.

A limited number of outcomes, in turn, must be juxtaposed onto the many different causes of intellectual disabilities. At last count, as many as 1000 different genetic anomalies were associated with intellectual disabilities (King et al. 2005). Although many of these conditions occur relatively infre-quently, genetic ID conditions still probably account for one-third or more of all individuals with intellectual disabilities (Matalainen et al. 1995). We thus have many causes and few outcomes or, to quote the clinical geneticist John Opitz (1985, p. 9), 'the causes are many, but the final developmental pathways are few.'

For our purposes, this pattern of many disorders but few outcomes leads to a more circumscribed approach. Sometimes, a genetic condition will be unique in some aspect of behaviour; it will more often be the case that an interesting behavioural outcome will not be unique but instead will be 'shared' with one or more other conditions. Such sharing is of interest itself and may be helpful in basic and applied fields.

BEHAVIOURAL ASPECTS THAT MAY POTENTIALLY BE UNIQUE TO A SINGLE SYNDROME

Given a more circumscribed search for behaviours that are unique to a single genetic disorder, where should one look? Although Flint and Yule (1994) were primarily interested in maladaptive behaviour and psychiatric conditions, one could search for unique behaviours in other domains. Consider, for example, a host of individual behaviours. Individuals with 5p- syndrome show a characteristic, high-pitched vocal cry, the 'cat cry' that led to the disorder's original name, cri-du-chat syndrome (Gersh et al. 1995). Individuals with Prader-Willi syndrome show extreme hyperphagia (Dykens 1999), leading to the motto of the Prader-Willi syndrome Association of the US (PWS-USA): 'Always hungry, never full.' Finally, individuals with Smith Magenis syndrome have been shown to have self-hugging behaviours (Finucane et al. 1994). In each case, the single genetic disorder shows a single, often maladaptive behaviour that is not seen to the same extent in any other genetic ID syndrome.

Individual behaviours are only one way in which total specificity can show itself. A second way involves profiles of cognitive, linguistic, or adaptive strengths and weaknesses. In this case, what is unique is not a single behaviour but instead a particular pattern of strengths and weaknesses.

Again, a few examples can be noted. In Williams syndrome, most individuals show a pattern in which linguistic abilities exceed visual-spatial abilities, a pattern that becomes more pronounced as individuals get older. In a longitudinal study examining individuals at six testings over a 4-year period, Jarrold et al. (2001) found that vocabulary age-equivalent scores (their measure of linguistic ability) were relatively strong compared to these same individuals' pattern construction age-equivalent scores (the measure of visual-spatial abilities). In addition, over the 4-year period, language levels increased more rapidly than did levels of visual-spatial skills. In essence, an already-existing strength became stronger as the child developed.

A similarly unique profile involves the ability of children with Prader-Willi syndrome to assemble jigsaw puzzles. Long considered a 'secondary criterion' of Prader-Willi syndrome (Holm et al. 1993), assembling jigsaw puzzles is a particular strength of children who have the deletion form of Prader-Willi syndrome. Children with the deletion form perform at or even above levels that one might expect for their chronological ages (Dykens 2002). Again, apart from children with Prader-Willi syndrome, no other genetic disorder shows such high puzzle-playing abilities, or abilities so far advanced relative to overall levels of cognitive functioning.

Finally, one can examine trajectories of development. Trajectories concern the rate of development at various ages during the child's life – the possibility that faster or slower development may occur at different ages. In various studies, boys with fragile-X syndrome seem to slow in their rates of development beginning in the adolescent years (Lachiewicz et al. 1987; Hodapp et al. 1990). Although such slowing is generally not found in children with mixed or heterogeneous causes for their mental retardation (Bernheimer & Keogh 1988; Stavrou 1990), slowing *per se* may not be unique to boys with fragile-X syndrome.

DOWN SYNDROME: UNIQUE OR NOT UNIQUE?

Given the definition, caveats and examples of total specificity, does DS show examples of unique individual behaviours, profiles, or trajectories? Let's examine each in turn.

INDIVIDUAL BEHAVIOURS

Compared to unique behaviours found in other syndromes, most individuals with DS do not seem to show any specific, individual behaviour that is unique. As noted above, the unique behaviours discovered so far include the cat-cry in 5p- syndrome, hyperphagia in Prader-Willi syndrome, and self-hugging in Smith Magenis syndrome. Each behaviour is seen in most persons with each syndrome, although not in all individuals (Dykens 1995). More importantly, these behaviours all involve fairly dramatic, often maladaptive behaviours.

Given more than 100 years of behavioural research on individuals with DS, it seems likely that any such salient behaviour would have been noticed. If present, such behaviours would have received comment by earlier observers, and later researchers would have conducted studies to examine these behaviours over time and in different situations. Although certain more subtle individual behaviours may have been missed, it seems prudent to conclude that few individual behaviours are unique to DS.

PROFILES

If only because DS has long shown several noteworthy areas of strength and weakness, unique profiles seem possible. Over many years of research, most individuals with DS have been shown to have deficits in expressive language and in grammar that are greater than their overall mental ages (Chapman & Hesketh 2000; Rondal 2005) as well as very high rates of problems with articulation (Leddy 1999). In contrast with individuals without disabilities, those with DS (on average) show better visual as compared with auditory short-term memories (Hodapp et al. 1999; Pueschel et al. 1986), a pattern that may become increasingly evident in the late teens (Hodapp & Ricci 2002).

Moreover, some profiles are being linked to underlying brain functioning. For many years, Nadel (1996, 1999) has argued that children with DS are deficient in tasks that use hippocampal functioning. Pennington et al. (2003) compared these children directly with MA-matched typically developing children on two sets of tasks. The first related to functioning of the prefrontal cortex, which involves holding information in active or working memory. The second examined hippocampal functioning, or the storage of episodic information in long-term memory. Although children with DS were equivalent on tasks relating to the prefrontal cortex, they performed more poorly than MA-matches on tasks involving the hippocampus.

There do, then, seem to be several different profiles of strengths and weaknesses that characterise most individuals with DS. It remains unclear whether such profiles are unique to DS or are found in other genetic conditions.

TRAJECTORIES

As in profiles, most individuals with DS show a particular trajectory of development. Examined over a many-year period, the highest IQ scores (a general measure of the rate of cognitive development) are found in the earliest years, with declining scores after that time.

Although reasons for such declining rates in intellectual development are unclear, a few explanations seem likely. One involves the ease or difficulty that children with DS have in achieving particular developmental tasks (Hodapp & Zigler 1990). For example, Dunst (1988, 1990) noted that infants with DS exhibited particular difficulties developing from Piaget's sensori-motor stage III to stage IV, and from stage IV to stage V. Similar difficulties may arise in negotiating the development of several stages of linguistic grammar. As Fowler et al. (1994) note, many children with DS have difficulties in accomplishing Brown's (1973) stage III grammar. Stage III grammar, lasting from roughly 30 to 36 months in typically developing children, features longer sentences that also include the correct usage of many grammatical morphemes ('-ed' for past tense, '-ing' for progressive tense); the beginnings of negatives, 'wh-' questions, and yes-no questions; and overgeneralisations such as 'feets' and 'goed'. Many children with DS remain at this developmental stage for many years. Rondal et al. (1988) found no correlation between chronological age and grammatical levels once children had reached stage III grammar. For children with DS, stage III grammar thus seems especially problematic and 'the slowdown at Stage III . . . raises the possibility that linguistic factors are one important determinant in explaining a child's failure to progress' (Fowler et al. 1994, p. 135).

Conversely, slowing may relate to certain as yet unspecified changes that relate more to the maturation of brain structures that are tied to the child's chronological age. Fowler (1988) notes that several of her children with Down syndrome simply did not develop in grammar from the ages of approximately 6 to 11 years. Before and after this time children developed but they showed a plateau in development during these middle childhood years (see also Gibson 1966). Together with their difficulties in mastering complex grammar and other aspects of language, such age-related slowing may further contribute to the slowing rates of development in these children as they grow older.

Without a better understanding of both how and when developmental slowing occurs for most children with DS, it remains unclear whether the slowing rates of development seen in DS are totally specific. From other studies, children with ID from heterogeneous causes do not slow in their rates of development as they grow older; 'slow but steady' development seems to be the norm (Stavrou 1990). In a few other groups (such as boys with fragile-X syndrome) slowing rates of development over age does hold. But the reasons for such slowing – whether it is related to difficulties in mastering specific tasks and/or to age-related neurological changes – remain unknown.

REMAINING BEHAVIOURAL ASPECTS IN DS

Two other behavioural aspects seem common to children with DS.

Fragility

One of the hallmarks of behavioural development in children with DS is its fragility. This term can have several meanings, but here it refers to the idea that children with DS more often show development that involves 'two steps forward, one step backward' and regressions are common. Intuitively, this more fragile developmental pattern would seem connected to – and might possibly even cause – some of the slowing developmental trajectories discussed above.

Before describing findings for children with DS, it is important to appreciate that regressions occur in the development of all children. Particularly during infancy, children often successfully perform a high-level task on one session but then fail the identical task on the next session several weeks later (Uzgiris 1987). Among children with DS, however, such backsliding occurs more often than in children without ID of the same levels of development. Compared to non-disabled children of the same mental ages, young children with DS show many more instances of regressions from one testing session to the next (Dunst 1990). Whereas infants and toddlers with DS showed regressions on over 17% of Uzgiris-Hunt scale items over five or six testings that were 3 to 5 weeks apart, non-DS infants averaged regression rates of only 7%. Such different percentages showed themselves across all sensorimotor domains, including object permanence, imitation, means-ends, causality and spatial relationships.

Additional evidence for fragility comes from adolescents and young adults with DS. In one study, Shepperdson (1995) examined two cohorts of British children with DS during infancy and again as teenagers (X = 16 years). Although slowing rates of development occurred in both cohorts, for both cohorts the best predictor of continued development was the level of stimulation provided to the teen or young adult. Even using a gross measure of level of stimulation, most outcomes related to level of environmental stimulation, usually accounting for 20–30% of the variance.

It appears, then, that more tentative, fragile advances characterise the development of children and young adults with DS. Although it remains unclear whether such fragility is unique to DS, it nevertheless seems important for the nature, amount and timing of interventions in this syndrome.

Sociability and Motivation

A second noteworthy aspect of behaviour in DS concerns sociability and motivation. For many years, researchers have debated the presence of a so-called 'DS personality', the possibility that most children with the disorder might have personalities that are more sociable and upbeat. Some researchers have argued that, on average, such a personality exists (Hodapp 1997) whereas others have argued against the presence of an aetiology-related personality (Wishart & Johnston 1990).

What seems less arguable is that children with DS, from very young ages, show high levels of socially oriented behaviours. Compared to typical children of the same mental ages, toddlers with DS, on average, spend more time looking to an interacting adult than to surrounding toys (Kasari et al. 1990). During the school-age years, these children remain more likely than others with intellectual disabilities to look to adults during problem-solving tasks (Kasari & Freeman 2001).

A further question concerns how children with DS use that sociability. In their study of preschoolers with DS, Pitcairn & Wishart (1994) noted that, 'The DS children were not simply more social. It was rather in their response to failure that they differed. They exploited their social skills, producing a variety of distracting behaviours that focused attention (their own and that of the experimenter) away from the task at hand' (p. 489).

In addition, children with DS seem to exploit such social distractors both before and after the toddler years. As Fidler (2005, in press) has shown, even infants with DS are developing in their use of social distractors. Later, during the school age years, children with DS again look to others, seemingly to avoid solving difficult problems (Kasari & Freeman 2001). However one comes down on the issue of a possible DS personality, these children are, as a group, fairly interested in interacting with others and some of those interactions are used to avoid performing difficult cognitive tasks.

REMAINING ISSUES

In reviewing the evidence concerning total specificity in the behaviour of children with DS, several major gaps become apparent. These include the following:

NEED FOR MORE AND BETTER STUDIES

To determine whether a specific behaviour, profile, or trajectory is unique to DS, we need studies that directly examine this issue. Until now, aetiology-based studies have almost always been lacking in their focus on this issue. As a result, we know that children with DS show particular profiles or trajectories over age but cannot determine the uniqueness of such behavioural characteristics.

Part of the problem relates to the need to progress beyond major behaviours. If indeed children with DS potentially show task- (or age-) related slowings, for example, we need studies that will examine this issue in DS versus other genetic aetiologies. Much of this work will need to first look closely at DS and then, in subsequent studies, examine specific, oftentimes subtle areas of strength and weakness to establish whether they are also found in children with other genetic syndromes.

NEED TO CONSIDER DEVELOPMENT

A second, related issue concerns development. Persons with different genetic syndromes are not born with all behaviours or profiles fully in place. In DS, too, the behavioural phenotype emerges over age. Fidler's work (this volume) exemplifies this search for DS behavioural profiles over the early years. Changes also emerge in the salience of strengths and weaknesses at older ages (Hodapp & Ricci 2002).

From this perspective, it is almost naïve to speak of behaviours or profiles that are unique to a specific aetiological group. Increasingly, we may need to go beyond the question of 'Is this behavioural characteristic unique to DS?' to ask instead 'Is this behavioural characteristic unique to children with DS who are of a specific age or specific level of functioning?' Individual behaviours, profiles and even slowing developmental trajectories seem dependent on the age or level of the child.

NEED TO TIE BOTH TO BRAIN CORRELATES AND TO INTERVENTION

Without ties to underlying brain mechanisms or to intervention, the search for unique behavioural characteristics becomes an academic exercise. Certain aspects of behaviour may – or may not – be unique, but the most important, interesting questions take this quest a step further.

Such next steps most likely go in two directions. A first direction ties to underlying brain functioning and structure. If a behavioural characteristic is unique to DS, what does this imply for connections to neurological functioning? Which structural or functional brain change(s) relate to any unique aspects of behaviour? Even non-unique behavioural aspects – those specific behaviours, profiles, or trajectories that are shared with one or more other syndromes – might also be examined in terms of 'brain-behaviour' connections.

Going in the opposite direction, what can we learn from unique aspects of DS behaviour for intervention? So far, aetiology-based behavioural interventions remain mostly unexamined, an unrealised dream. Although recommendations for aetiology-based interventions have been made for several groups, such suggestions remain unexamined (Hodapp & Fidler 1999; Hodapp et al. 2003).

Given the major advances of aetiology-based behavioural research since the mid-1980s, we are on the edge of a new frontier, a border that remains uncrossed as it relates to many aspects of aetiology-related behaviours. As this chapter illustrates, children with DS do exhibit certain aetiology-related profiles and trajectories, although we still do not know whether such profiles and trajectories are unique to this syndrome alone. We also do not yet know the specific brain correlates or intervention implications of such aetiology-related aspects of behaviour. In short, although we have advanced greatly in recent years in understanding aetiology-related behaviours in this and other genetic ID syndromes, we continue to have a long way to go.

REFERENCES

Achenbach, T. M. (1991) *Manual for the Child Behaviour Checklist – 4–18 – and 1991 Profiles.* Burlington VT: University of Vermont.

Anderson, M. (2001) Conceptions of intelligence. *J Child Psychol Psychiat,* **42,** 287–298.

Bernheimer, L. C., Keogh, B. (1988) Stability of cognitive performance of children with developmental delays. *Am J Ment Retard,* **92,** 539–542.

Brown, R. (1973) *A First Language.* Cambridge MA: Harvard University Press.

Chapman, R. J., Hesketh, L. J. (2000) Behavioural phenotype of individuals with Down syndrome. *Mental Retardation and Developmental Disorders Research Reviews,* **6,** 84–95.

Costa, P. T., McCrae R. R. (1992) The 5-factor model of personality and its relevance to personality disorders. *J Pers Disord,* **6,** 343–359.

Costa, P. T., McCrae, R. R. (1997) Personality trait structure as a human universal. *Am Psychol,* **52,** 509–516.

Dunst, C. J. (1988) Stage transitioning in the sensorimotor development of Down's syndrome infants. *J Ment Defic Res,* **32,** 405–410.

Dunst, C. J. (1990) Sensorimotor development of infants with Down syndrome. In D. Cicchetti, M. Beeghly (eds) (1990) *Children with Down Syndrome: A Developmental Approach.* Cambridge UK: Cambridge University Press, pp. 180–230.

Dykens, E. M. (1995) Measuring behavioural phenotypes: provocations from the 'new genetics.' Am J Ment Retard 99, 522–532.

Dykens, E. M. (1999) Prader-Willi syndrome. In H. Tager-Flusberg (ed.) *Neurodevelopmental Disorders.* Cambridge MA: MIT Press, pp. 137–154.

Dykens, E. M. (2002) Are jigsaw puzzles 'spared' in persons with Prader-Willi syndrome? *J Child Psychol Psychiatr,* **43,** 343–352.

Fidler, D. J. (2005) The emerging Down syndrome behavioural phenotype in early childhood. *Infants and Young Children,* **18,** 86–103.

Fidler, D. J. (in press) Motivation and etiology-specific cognitive-linguistic profiles. *International Review of Research in Mental Retardation.*

Finucane, B. M., Konar, D., Haas-Givler, B., Kurtz, M. D., Scott, L. I. (1994) The spasmodic upper-body squeeze: a characteristic behaviour in Smith-Magenis syndrome. *Dev Med Child Neurol*, **36**, 78–83.

Flint, J., Yule, W. (1994) Behavioural phenotypes. In M. Rutter, E. Taylor, L. Hersov (eds) *Child and Adolescent Psychiatry: Modern Approaches*, 3rd edn. London: Blackwell Scientific, pp. 666–687.

Fowler, A. E. (1988) Determinants of rate of language growth in children with DS. In L. Nadel (ed.) *The Psychobiology of Down Syndrome*. Cambridge MA: MIT Press, pp. 217–245.

Fowler, A. E. Gelman, R., Gleitman, L. R. (1994) The course of language learning in children with Down syndrome. In H. Tager-Flusberg (ed.) *Constraints on Language Acquisition: Studies of Atypical Children*. Hillsdale NJ: Erlbaum.

Gersh, M., Goodart, S. A., Pasztor, L. M., Harris, D. J., Weiss, L., Overhauser, J. (1995) Evidence for a distinct region causing a cat-like cry in patients with 5p- deletions. *Am J Hum Genet*, **56**, 1404–1410.

Gibson, D. (1966) Early developmental staging as a prophesy index in Down's syndrome. *Am J Ment Defic*, **70**, 825–828.

Gibson, D. (1978) *Down's Syndrome: The Psychology of Mongolism*. Cambridge UK: Cambridge University Press.

Hodapp, R. M. (1997) Direct and indirect behavioural effects of different genetic disorders of mental retardation. *Am J Ment Retard*, **102**, 67–79.

Hodapp, R. M., DesJardin, J. L., Ricci, L. A. (2003) Genetic syndromes of mental retardation: should they matter for the early interventionist? *Infants and Young Children*, **16**, 152–160.

Hodapp, R. M., Dykens, E. M. (2004) Studying behavioural phenotypes: Issues, benefits, challenges. In E. Emerson, C. Hatton, T. Parmenter, T. Thompson (eds) *International Handbook of Applied Research in Intellectual Disabilities*. New York: John Wiley & Sons, pp. 203–220.

Hodapp, R. M., Dykens, E. M., Hagerman, R., Schreiner, R., Lachiewicz, A., Leckman, J. F. (1990) Developmental implications of changing trajectories of IQ in males with fragile X syndrome. *Journal of the American Academy of Child and Adolescent Psychiatry*, **29**, 214–219.

Hodapp, R. M., Evans, D., Gray, F. L. (1999) Intellectual development in children with Down syndrome. In J. A. Rondal, J. Perera, L. Nadel (eds) *Down's Syndrome: A Review of Current Knowledge*. London: Whurr Publishers, pp. 124–132.

Hodapp, R. M., Fidler, D. J. (1999) Special education and genetics: connections for the 21st century. *J Spec Educ*, **33**, 130–137.

Hodapp, R. M., Ricci, L. A. (2002) Behavioural phenotypes and educational practice: the unrealized connection. In G. O'Brien (eds) Behavioural Phenotypes in Clinical Practice. London: Mac Keith Press, pp. 137–151.

Hodapp, R. M., Zigler, E. (1990) Applying the developmental perspective to children with Down syndrome. In D. Cicchetti, M. Beeghly (eds) *Children with Down Syndrome: A Developmental Perspective*. New York: Cambridge University Press, pp. 1–28.

Holm, V. A., Cassidy, S. B., Butler, M. G., Hanchett, J. M., Greenswag, L. R., Whitman, B. Y., et al. (1993) Prader-Willi syndrome: consensus diagnostic criteria. *Pediatrics*, **91**, 398–402.

Jarrold, C., Baddeley, A. D., Hewes, A. K., Phillips, C. (2001) A longitudinal assessment of diverging verbal and non-verbal abilities in the Williams syndrome phenotype. *Cortex*, **37**, 423–431.

Kasari, C., Freeman, S. F. N. (2001) Task-related social behaviour in children with Down syndrome. *Am J Ment Retard*, **106**, 253–264.

Kasari, C., Mundy, P., Yirmiya, N., Sigman, M. (1990) Affect and attention in children with Down syndrome. *Am J Ment Retard*, **95**, 55–67.

King, B. H., Hodapp, R. M., Dykens, E. M. (2005) Mental retardation. In H. I. Kaplan, B. J. Sadock (eds) *Comprehensive Textbook of Psychiatry*, 8th edn. Vol. 2. Baltimore: Williams & Wilkins, pp. 3076–3106.

Lachiewicz, A. M., Guiollion, C., Spridigliozzi, G., Aylsworth, A. (1987) Declining IQs of young males with fragile X syndrome. *Am J Ment Retard*, **92**, 272–278.

Leddy, M. (1999) The biological bases of speech in people with Down syndrome. In J. F. Miller, M. Leddy, L. A. Leavitt (eds) *Improving the Communication of People with Down Syndrome*. Baltimore: Paul H. Brookes Co, pp. 60–80.

Matalainen, R., Airaksinen, E., Mononen, T., Launiala, K., Kaarianen, R. (1995) A population-based study of the causes of severe and profound mental retardation. *Acta Pediatrica*, **84**, 261–266.

Nadel, L. (1996) Learning, memory, and neural functioning in Down's syndrome. In J. A. Rondal, J. Perera, L. Nadel, A. Comblain (eds) *Down's Syndrome: Psychological, Psychobiological, and Soci-educational Perspectives*. London: Whurr Publishers, pp. 21–42.

Nadel, L. (1999) Learning and memory in Down syndrome. In J. A. Rondal, J. Perera, L. Nadel (eds) *Down Syndrome: A Review of Current Knowledge*. London: Whurr Publishers, pp. 133–142.

Opitz, J. M. (1985) Editorial comment: the developmental field concept. *Am J Med Genet*, **21**, 1–11.

Pennington, B., Moon, J., Edgin, J., Stedron J., Nadel, L. (2003). The neuropsychology of DS: evidence for hippocampal dysfunction. *Child Development*, **74**, 75–93.

Pennington, B., O'Connor, R., Sudhalter, V. (1991) Toward a neuropsychology of fragile X syndrome. In R. J. Hagerman, A. C. Silverman (eds) *Fragile X Syndrome: Diagnosis, Treatment, and Research*. Baltimore: Johns Hopkins University Press, pp. 173–201.

Pitcairn, T. K., Wishart, J. G. (1994) Reactions of young children with Down syndrome to an impossible task. *Br J Dev Psychol*, **12**, 485–489.

Pueschel, S. R., Gallagher, P. L., Zartler, A. S., Pezzullo, J. C. (1986) Cognitive and learning profiles in children with Down syndrome. *Res Dev Disabil*, **8**, 21–37.

Rondal, J. A. (2005) Intersyndrome and intrasyndrome language differences. In J. A. Rondal, R. M. Hodapp, S. Soresi, E. M. Dykens, L. Nota (eds) *Intellectual Disabilities: Genetics, Behaviour, and Inclusion*. London: Whurr Publishers, pp. 49–113.

Rondal, J. A., Ghiotto, M., Bredart, S., Bachelet, J.-F. (1988) Mean length of utterance of children with Down syndrome. *Am J Ment Retard*, **93**, 64–66.

Shepperdson, B. (1995) Two longitudinal studies of the abilities of people with Down's syndrome. *J Intellect Disabil Res*, **39**, 419–431.

Stavrou, E. (1990) The long-term stability of WISC-R scores in mildly retarded and learning disabled children. *Psychol Schools*, **27**, 101–110.

Uzgiris, I. C. (1987) The study of sequential order in cognitive development. In I. C. Uzgiris, J. McV. Hunt (eds) *Infant Performance and Experience*. Urbana-Champaign IL: University of Illinois Press, pp. 129–167.

Wagner, S., Ganiban, J. M., Cicchetti, D. (1990) Attention, memory, and perception in infants with Down syndrome: review and commentary. In D. Cicchetti, M. Beeghly (eds) *Children with Down Syndrome: A Developmental Perspective*. Cambridge: Cambridge University Press, pp. 147–179.

Wishart, J. G., Johnston, F. H. (1990) The effects of experience on attribution of a stereotyped personality to children with Down's syndrome. *Journal of Intellectual Disability Research*, **34**, 409–420.

9 The Emergence of a Syndrome-specific Personality Profile in Young Children with Down Syndrome

DEBORAH J. FIDLER
Colorado State University, Fort Collins, USA

SUMMARY

For decades, researchers and practitioners have attempted to find evidence for a personality stereotype in individuals with Down syndrome (DS) that includes a pleasant, affectionate, and passive behaviour style. However, a more nuanced exploration of personality and motivation in DS reveals complexity beyond this pleasant stereotype, including reports of a less persistent motivational orientation and overreliance on social behaviours during cognitively challenging tasks. It is hypothesised that the personality-motivation profile observed in individuals with DS emerges as a result of the cross-domain relations between more primary (cognitive, social-emotional) aspects of the DS behavioural phenotype. If this is true, it might be possible to alter the developmental trajectory of this personality-motivation profile with targeted and time-sensitive intervention. Implications for intervention planning are discussed.

INTRODUCTION

Many areas of the Down syndrome behavioural phenotype have been well researched, with strengths and weaknesses identified in information processing, social functioning, motor development, and language (Byrne et al. 1995; Fidler et al. 2005b; Gibbs & Thorpe 1983; Hesketh & Chapman 1998; Jarrold & Baddeley 1997; Jarrold, Baddeley & Hewes 1999; Jobling 1998; Klein & Mervis 1999; Laws 1998; Miller & Leddy 1999; Mon-Williams

Down Syndrome: Neurobehavioural Specificity. Edited by JA Rondal and J Perera.
© 2006 John Wiley & Sons Ltd.

et al. 2001; Rodgers 1987; Rosner et al. 2004; Sigman & Ruskin 1999; Wishart & Johnston 1990; Wang & Bellugi 1994).

Another area of potential importance in the DS behavioural phenotype relates to the personality-motivational style. For decades, researchers and practitioners have attempted to describe commonalities in personality style among individuals with DS, with some arguing for a stereotype involving a pleasant, affectionate and passive personality style (Gibbs & Thorpe 1983; Rodgers 1987). This stereotype has been supported by studies of parent perception of children with Down syndrome where, in one study, over 50% of 11-year-old children with DS were described as 'affectionate', 'loveable', 'nice' and 'getting on well with other people' (Carr 1995). A large percentage of the children in this study were also described as 'cheerful', 'generous' and 'fun' (Carr 1995). There are also reports of increased positive mood and predictability in behaviour in individuals with Down syndrome, supporting the more positive pleasant aspects of the personality stereotype, as well as reports of lower activity levels, less persistence, and more distractibility in than other children, supporting the more passive aspects of the stereotype (Gunn & Cuskelly, 1991).

However, a more nuanced exploration of personality-motivation in Down syndrome reveals great complexity in personality development and motivational style over time. In addition to these positive perceptions of personality in individuals with Down syndrome, other research reports have described individuals with Down syndrome as showing a specific motivational orientation involving lower levels of task persistence and higher levels of off-task social behaviours (Landry & Chapieski 1990; Pitcairn & Wishart 1994; Ruskin et al. 1994; Vlachou & Farrell 2000; Kasari & Freeman 2001). This lowered persistence is sometimes complemented by a stubborn or strong-willed personality streak, also described in studies of temperament in Down syndrome (Gibson 1978; Carr 1995).

Although they have not received the same amount of attention from researchers as more positive personality dimensions, poor persistence and a stubborn temperament may have far-reaching implications for developmental outcomes in DS. Some researchers suggest that these characteristics contribute to some of the inconsistency in developmental performances observed in young children with DS. Several studies have reported that young children with DS aged 6 months to 4 years show significant regressions on the same testing battery across sessions (Morss 1983; Wishart & Duffy 1990) and it has been noted that many of these regressions result from children's refusal to engage in tasks (Wishart & Duffy 1990; Pitcairn & Wishart 1994).

In fact this phenomenon has been quantified by researchers interested in exploring motivational performance in children with DS. Jennifer Wishart and her colleagues have observed that when faced with cognitive challenges in laboratory settings, children with DS often avoid tasks with both positive and negative behaviours more frequently than other children (Wishart 1996).

In young children, these behaviours can include refusing to look at a task, struggling out of a chair, or sudden crying behaviour (Wishart & Bower 1984). Older children have been shown to engage experimenters with off-task social behaviour that distracts them from the task at hand (Pitcairn & Wishart 1994). These social behaviours might include directing the experimenter's attention to something else and/or using 'party trick' behaviours such as clapping hands. Wishart (1996) describes these 'cognitive avoidant' or 'quitting out' behaviours as a unique feature in the performance of children with DS on developmental assessments.

Beyond the implications for assessment in research settings, it may be that this weak motivational orientation affects other areas of functioning in DS, including performance in educational and intervention settings. Wishart (1996) argues that, '[f]rom a very early age, it would appear that the Down syndrome children are avoiding opportunities for learning new skills, making poor use of skills that are acquired, and failing to consolidate skills into their repertoires' (Wishart 1996). If this is true, then understanding personality-motivational orientation in individuals with DS may offer researchers a unique opportunity to improve the effectiveness of intervention and educational programming in individuals with DS. This may hold for educational programming in school settings for children and adolescents who have already developed this profile and it may especially be relevant in early intervention settings where it may be possible to try to prevent this profile from ever emerging. In order to plan effective intervention it may be important to understand how this personality profile comes to be.

EXPLORING THE ORIGINS OF THE PERSONALITY-MOTIVATION PROFILE IN DOWN SYNDROME

How does this personality profile involving positive mood and sociability coupled with lowered persistence and 'quitting out' behaviours emerge and develop over time? Unlike other aspects of the DS behavioural phenotype, which may have their origins in the intersection between genetics and brain development (for example, stronger visual processing and weaker verbal processing – see Pueschel et al. 1987; Wang & Bellugi 1994; Frangou et al. 1997; Jarrold et al. 1999; Klein & Mervis 1999; Laws 1998; Pinter et al. 2001) it might be that this personality profile emerges as a 'secondary phenotypic' outcome. That is, the personality-motivation profile observed in individuals with DS may emerge as a result of the cross-domain relations between more primary (cognitive, social-emotional) aspects of the Down syndrome behavioural phenotype.

In the following sections we will explore the intersection between early strengths in social functioning and deficits in cognition and means-end thinking and how, together, they may contribute to the emergence of a personality profile that involves an overreliance on an endearing social style at the expense of a more persistent motivational orientation. We first explore two 'primary phenotypic' behavioural outcomes associated with early development in Down syndrome: the early cognitive phenotype and the early social-emotional phenotype. We will then explore the cross-domain relations between social and cognitive functioning that may predispose children with Down syndrome to adopt the specific personality-motivation style often observed in this population.

PRIMARY PHENOTYPIC OUTCOMES: COGNITION

In typically developing infants, one of the most important early cognitive achievements is the development of means-end, or instrumental thinking (Piaget 1952; Bjorklund 2000). Means-end thinking begins to develop during the first 2 to 8 months of life. In its earliest forms, means-end thinking generally involves linking a chain of behaviours together as a means to reach an end state, such as pulling on a string to obtain a toy that is attached to the string. For example, typically developing 2- to 8-month-old infants show contingency learning skills that involve learning to move certain body parts (such as pulling their arm) as a means to achieving reinforcement outcomes (picture displays and music – Lewis et al. 1990). At approximately 8 months, infants discover how manual skills may be used to achieve new goals. New behaviours, such as reaching and grasping, open up a whole set of different goals and these new strategies are used as a means to achieve desired end states.

However, the existing literature on the development of means-end thinking in infants and toddlers with Down syndrome suggests that this is an area of major challenge. In a study of contingency learning (an early version of cause and effect/means-end thinking), 3-month-old infants with Down syndrome showed equivalent performances to typical infants on contingent learning tasks that involved reinforcement for their own leg kicking, including equivalent initial learning, learning speed, and retention (Ohr & Fagen 1991). However, the same research team (Ohr & Fagen 1994) reported that by 9 months, the same cohort of infants with DS demonstrated significantly impaired contingency learning relative to typically developing infants. The authors of this series of studies suggested that there is a decline in contingency learning and conditionability in infants with DS over the first year of life. If means-end thinking relies in part on contingency learning, this could be early evidence of atypical development of means-end thinking that is specific to the population of infants with DS.

Further evidence for atypical development of instrumental thinking can be found in a study of sensorimotor stage transitioning in infants with Down syndrome (Uzgiris & Hunt 1979). Dunst (1988) found that infants with

Down syndrome take longer to move from means-end stage V (for example, pulling a string to obtain a toy) to means-end stage VI (for example, showing intention while putting a necklace in a cup) than typically developing infants. But this slower stage transitioning was not evident in other areas, such as object permanence, gestural imitation and causality. Delays in the emergence of more advanced means-end thinking in infancy may be evidence of specific impairments in aspects of problem solving skills in DS.

Means-end thinking has also been found to be unrelated to other domains of sensorimotor development, including object permanence, vocal imitation, gestural imitation, operational causality, spatial relationships, and object schemes in infants with Down syndrome (Dunst & Rheingrover 1983). This is evidence of a lack of stage congruence between means-end performance and performances in these other aspects of sensorimotor functioning. Others report no associations between means-end performances at 5 months and later at 13, 15, 18, and 24 months in infants with DS (Cicchetti et al. 1987). In contrast, strong associations are observed in other sensorimotor areas, such as vocal imitation, object permanence, and spatial relations. These findings suggest that while many other areas of sensorimotor functioning develop in concert with one another in DS, means-end thinking follows an atypical and slower developmental trajectory.

Beyond infancy, there is also indirect evidence that young children with DS show continued delays in the means-end (instrumental) component of problem solving. Ruskin et al. (1994) reported that toddlers with DS in their study showed significantly shorter chains of continuous goal-directed mastery behaviours with a cause-and-effect toy (for example, fitting blocks through corresponding holes) than MA-matched typically developing children. This suggests that toddlers with DS continue to have difficulty putting together chains of behaviour as a means to reaching a particular end. Similarly, our team (Fidler et al. 2005a) found that toddlers with DS showed less optimal strategies on an object retrieval problem-solving task (obtaining a desired item from under a plastic box) than MA-matched typically developing toddlers and toddlers with other developmental disabilities.

Thus, deficits in the building blocks of instrumental or strategic thinking have been observed from the earliest stages of the development of means-end thinking and in many different types of laboratory settings. But the impact of these findings may go beyond observing performances on instrumental tasks in laboratory settings. Young children with DS display lower levels of causality pleasure, showing fewer positive facial displays during goal-directed mastery behaviours than the comparison group of typically developing children (Ruskin et al. 1994). This suggests that children with DS not only display deficits in instrumental thinking but they also do not show usual amount of enjoyment and pleasure when engaging in tasks that involve means-end or strategic thinking. This may have important implications for developing a motivational orientation that involves engaging with new and challenging tasks.

PRIMARY PHENOTYPIC OUTCOMES: SOCIAL FUNCTIONING

Delays in the development of instrumental thinking in young children with DS are complemented by an emerging relative strength in social-emotional functioning. By the time they reach the age of 3 years, many children with DS already show quantifiable strengths in social functioning as measured by the Vineland Adaptive Behavior Scales (Fidler et al., in press b). Our team has also reported that early orienting and engagement behaviours in young children with DS may be a specific area of developmental competence that grows at a faster pace than others areas of development (such as emotion regulation or motor functioning). While some studies report no significant temperament differences between infants with Down syndrome and typical infants (Ohr & Fagen 1994; Vaughn et al. 1994), other studies report that young children with DS are of more positive mood, more rhythmic and less intense than CA-matched children (Gunn & Berry 1985).

There is also evidence of emerging areas of competence within some aspects of social functioning in infancy in DS. Early looking behaviour (Crown et al. 1992; Gunn et al. 1982), vocalizing (Legerstee, Bowman & Fels 1992), and facial imitation in infancy (Heiman & Ullstadius 1999) have been identified as evidence of social relatedness in the first year of life. Although the onset of looking behaviour (at parent) is delayed during the first few months of development, by the middle of the first year, infants with DS may show increased looking behaviour toward their parent relative to other infants (Crown et al. 1992; Gunn et al. 1982). Three issues are notable in these behavioural findings. First, these behaviours may be evidence of the competent achievement of primary intersubjective milestones in infancy, wherein infants with DS develop behaviours that are evidence of core social relatedness; but these strengths may not translate into competence in all areas of subsequent social development. Second, looking behaviour for social purposes does not seem to translate into looking behaviour for instrumental purposes, as young children with DS show lesser amounts of social referencing than other children at similar developmental levels (Kasari et al. 1995; Walden et al. 1991). Third, while many young children with DS show these early behaviours, there is a subgroup of children who do not, and these children may present with comorbid psychiatric diagnoses, such as autism.

Some aspects of social behaviour in toddlers and preschoolers with DS also seem to develop with competence. Young children with DS show appropriate levels of joint attention for their developmental level (Mundy et al. 1988; Sigman & Ruskin 1999), more play acts than other children at similar developmental levels (Sigman & Ruskin 1999), and they attend to the emotional signals (Sigman & Ruskin 1999) and initiations of others (Bressanutti, Sachs & Mahoney 1992). In terms of attachment, there is some disagreement regarding whether children with DS show higher levels of insecure attachment (Berry, Gunn & Andrews 1980; Vaughn et al. 1994), although questions have been raised regarding the appropriateness of the 'strange situation' paradigm for children with developmental delays.

In addition to the development of core relatedness behaviours in young children with DS, there may be some uniqueness to the development of emotional displays as well. By the time they reach middle childhood, children with DS show more frequent smiling behaviour than other children with developmental disabilities (Fidler, Barrett & Most 2005a). Infants with DS were originally thought to show more muted emotional signalling relative to other infants (Berger & Cunningham 1986; Buckhalt, Rutherford & Goldberg 1978; Cicchetti & Sroufe 1978). However, more frequent muted signals seem to happen in the context of appropriate levels of high intensity smiles (Kasari et al. 1990; Knieps et al. 1994). This suggests that there may be increased positive emotional signalling during the earliest years of development in young children with DS as well.

Finally, our team has also recently reported emerging competence in social functioning in the form of faster developmental rates in certain areas. In one study where infants with DS were assessed with the Bayley Scales of Infant Development at 12 and the 30 months, children with DS made greater gains in the Orientation/Engagement domains than they did in other domains including cognition and motor functioning (Fidler et al. 2005b). In addition, growth in the orientation/engagement domain of the Bayley was significantly more rapid in the DS group than in an MA-matched group of children with idiopathic developmental delays. At Time 1, children in both groups showed mean percentile scores in the 37th percentile. However, by Time 2, the DS group showed mean percentile scores in the 58th percentile (SD = 13.32), while mean comparison group scores showed an average in the 42nd percentile (SD = 18.85). This is an average gain of 20 percentile points in the DS group. In comparison, the gains made by the comparison group children were more modest – a mean change of roughly 5 percentile points, which is approximately 15 percentile points or 75% less than the mean gain made by the DS group.

In addition, within-individual comparisons in this study suggested that greater gains were observed in orientation/engagement scores in comparison with other aspects of social-emotional functioning, such as performance in the emotion regulation domain of the Bayley. This suggests that the early strengths in social-emotional functioning are not domain general but may be specific to the development of some aspects of primary intersubjectivity. Taken together, findings from this recent study contribute to larger body of literature supporting the notion that early orienting and engagement behaviours in young children with DS may be a specific area of developmental competence that grows at a faster pace than other areas of development. It is important to note, however, that later social development may not continue with such strength as the cognitive demands on social functioning increase.

Young children with DS seem to show a general profile of delays in the development of instrumental thinking, coupled with emerging relative strengths in social-emotional functioning. In the next section, we explore an example of the manifestation of the difference in social versus instrumental competence in young children with DS: a split between requesting and joint attention behaviours in toddlers with DS.

SOCIAL/INSTRUMENTAL SPLIT IN THE EMERGENCE OF INTENTIONAL COMMUNICATION IN DS

As early cognitive and social skills are emerging, they intersect with the development of nonverbal communication skills. When typically developing infants reach the ages of 9 to 13 months they begin to use intentional communication in the form of joint attention and requesting. However, an important difference is observed in the nature of intentional communication in children with DS versus typically developing children or even other children with developmental disabilities. This difference relates to the emergence of nonverbal communication for social purposes and the emergence of nonverbal communication for instrumental purposes (as a means to an end).

Several studies have shown that early nonverbal social communication behaviours (such as joint attention) emerge as a relative strength in young children with DS, whereas early nonverbal instrumental communication behaviours (such as requesting) emerge as an area of relative weakness (Mundy et al. 1988; Wetherby et al. 1989; Fidler et al., in press c). For example, our team showed significantly fewer overall instrumental requests and low-level instrumental requests than a group of MA-matched typically developing infants and toddlers on the Early Social Communication Scales (Fidler et al., in press c). A split between instrumental gesturing (gesturing as a means to an end) and social gesturing (gesturing for the sake of social sharing) was evidenced in the dissociation between nonverbal requesting and joint attention skills in the DS group.

However, it is interesting to note that this requesting deficit seemed to be specific to instrumental requesting situations in our study (Fidler et al., in press c). In fact, young children with DS in our study showed marginally more requests during social routines. This suggests that the deficit in requesting in DS did not result from difficulties with performing specific acts associated with requesting (eye contact or reaching) but may have to do with using those behaviours as a means to an end and regulating another's behaviour for instrumental purposes. Moreover, our study reported an association between instrumental requesting behaviour and problem solving perform-ances in the young children with DS group. This suggests that the deficit in requesting behaviour previously reported in toddlers with DS might be a function of poor means-end functioning and not deficits in communication.

CROSS-DOMAIN RELATIONS

Thus, there is evidence that the earliest years of life for many individuals with DS involve emerging strength in social functioning (including strengths in the emergence of nonverbal social communication) and deficits in the development of means-end or strategic thinking (including deficits in the emergence of nonverbal instrumental communication). It is hypothesised here that the cross-domain relations between these two developing areas of functioning contribute to the emergence of a specific personality-motivation orientation, including poorer persistence and an over-reliance on social strategies.

Poorer persistence could be the indirect result of emerging difficulties with instrumental and strategic thinking during infancy in DS. Toddlers and pre-schoolers with DS who quit out of tasks or abandon challenging situations may be doing so because they are simply not able to generate new, more viable strategies to complete the task. That is, they have difficulty coming up with different options that serve as a means to the end of completing the task. Thus, a more passive and less persistent personality-motivation style could be directly linked to emerging primary deficits in instrumental reasoning and in cognition more generally.

Furthermore, in those instances when children with DS are not able to generate new strategies that can serve as a means to an end, it might be that what comes most naturally to them is to recruit their strengths in social skills. As a result, they may develop a style that involves responding to chal-lenging situations with charming or socially engaging behaviours that, ultimately, take them (and their social partner) off task. Or, they might rely on another social strategy, such as recruiting a social partner to help them complete a task, which has also been demonstrated in several laboratory studies (Kasari & Freeman 2001; Fidler et al. 2005a). In either case, the coupling of poor strategic thinking and strengths in social relatedness is hypothesised to lead to the less persistent and overly social personality-motivational orientation observed in this population. Even in the cases when social strategies are not selected, rather than generating a new strategy for resolving a problem at hand, stubborn behaviour suggests that children with DS become stuck on one particular strategy or approach and cannot become 'unstuck' from it.

If it is true that a less persistent motivational orientation emerges as a secondary phenotypic result of more primary strengths in social functioning and deficits in instrumental (means-end) thinking, it might be possible to alter the developmental trajectory of this personality-motivation profile with targeted and time-sensitive intervention. For example, it might be possible to focus on strengthening early means-end or strategic thinking in very young children with DS in order to prevent the deceleration of these skills, which leads to a split in social and instrumental functioning by the time that intentional communication emerges. Addressing the development of instrumental thinking at this early stage may help to promote a more adaptive personality-motivation style in later early childhood and beyond.

There are several potential ways to approach this type of intervention. For example, it may be possible to strengthen means-end thinking by targeting early instrumental requesting behaviour when a toddler with DS reaches the mental age of 9–13 months. This approach may be particularly preferable in that it is mediated by social signalling, thus making it a more learnable entry point than targeting cause and effect thinking through toys or other non-social stimuli. It may also be possible to shape different instrumental requesting signals to encourage flexibility and generalisability across various situations. Although targeting requesting in young children with DS remains only a hypothetical entry point, there is evidence mounting at this point to suggest that, at the very least, this may be a potentially effective entry-point for intervention.

Another important area for intervention may relate to the strengthening of behaviour chaining in young children with DS. There is evidence that young children with DS do not effectively chain sequences of goal-directed behaviours during play and non-social instrumental tasks (Ruskin et al. 1994). It may be that strategising difficulties are compounded by the cognitive load involved in chaining together a sequence of behaviours.

Often, more difficult real-life problem-solving tasks involve performing more than one behaviour in a sequence in order to solve the problem effectively (for example, find keys, select appropriate key, unlock door). Ideas for intervention to strengthen these skills are likely to be useful, constructing easy-to-solve problem-solving tasks that require more than one step and encouraging practice in assisted settings.

In exploring the origins of the personality-motivation orientation in individuals with DS, it may be possible to preserve the more positive aspects of the profile (social motivation), while targeting the maladaptive aspects of the profile (quitting-out behaviour). Although the suggested techniques remain unproven by empirical studies at this time, continued research in this area may yield more definitive support for these suggestions. Even given this caveat, it is likely that promoting better motivational development in individuals with DS with targeted and time-sensitive techniques will be effective and may affect development beyond simply improving adaptation.

Helping young children with DS to recognise their own ability to generate effective strategies may lead to improved instrumental functioning and may serve to improve academic performance, independence skills and outcomes in adulthood.

REFERENCES

Berger, J., Cunningham, C. C. (1986) Aspects of early social smiling by infants with Down's syndrome. *Child Care Health Dev*, **12**, 13–24.

Berry, P., Gunn, P., Andrews, R. (1980) Behavior of Down syndrome infants in a strange situation. *Am J Ment Defic*, **85**, 213–218.

Bjorklund, D. F. (2000) *Children's Thinking: Developmental Function and Individual Differences*. Belmont CA: Wadsworth.

Bressanutti, L., Sachs, J., Mahoney, G. (1992) Predictors of young children's compliance to maternal behavior requests. *International Journal of Cognitive Education and Mediated Learning*, **2**, 198–209.

Buckhalt, J. A., Rutherford, R. B., Goldberg, K. E. (1978) Verbal and nonverbal interaction of mothers with their Down's syndrome and nonretarded infants. *Am J Ment Defic*, **82**, 337–343.

Byrne, A., Buckley, S., MacDonald, J., Bird, G. (1995) Investigating the literacy, language, and memory skills of children with Down's syndrome. *Down's Syndrome: Research and Practice*, **3**, 53–58.

Carr, J. (1995) *Down's Syndrome: Children Growing Up*. Cambridge: Cambridge University Press.

Cicchetti, D., Mans-Wagener, L. (1987) Sequences, stages, and structures in the organization of cognitive development in infants with Down syndrome. In I. C. Uzgiris, J. M. Hunt, (eds) *Infant Performance and Experience: New Findings with the Ordinal Scales*. Urbana: University of Illinois Press, pp. 281–310.

Cicchetti, D., Sroufe, L. A. (1978) An organizational view of affect: Illustration from the study of Down's syndrome infants. In M. Lewis, L. A. Rosenbaum (eds) *The Development of Affect*. New York: Plenum Press.

Crown, C. L., Feldstein, S., Jasnow, M. D., Beebe, B. (1992) Down's syndrome and infant gaze: gaze behavior of Down's syndrome and nondelayed infants in interactions with their mothers. *Eur J Child Adolesc Psychiatr: Acta Paedopsychiatrica*, **55**, 51–55.

Dunst, C. (1988) Stage transitioning in the sensorimotor development in Down's syndrome infants. *J Ment Defic Res*, **32**, 405–410.

Dunst, C., Rheingrover, R. M. (1983) Structural characteristics of sensorimotor development among Down's syndrome infants. *J Ment Defic Res*, **27**, 11–22.

Fidler, D. J., Barrett, K. C., Most, D. E. (in press, a) Age-related differences in smiling and personality in Down syndrome. *J Dev Phys Disabil*.

Fidler, D. J., Hepburn, S., Mankin, G., & Rogers, S. (2005a). Praxis skills in young children with Down syndrome, other developmental disabilities, and typically developing children. *Am J Occup Ther*, **59**, 129–138.

Fidler, D. J., Hepburn, S., Rogers, S. (in press, b) Early learning and adaptive behavior in toddlers with Down syndrome: Evidence for an emerging behavioral phenotype? *Down Syndrome: Research and Practice*.

Fidler, D. J., Most, D. E., Booth-LaForce, C., Kelly, J. (2005b) Emerging social strengths in young children with Down syndrome at 12 and 30 months. Manuscript under review.

Fidler, D. J., Philofsky, A., Hepburn, S. L., Rogers, S. J. (in press, c) Nonverbal requesting and problem solving in young children with Down syndrome. *Am J Ment Retard*.

Frangou, S., Aylward, E., Warren, A., Sharma, T., Barta, P., Pearlson, G. (1997) Small planum temporale volume in Down's syndrome: a volumetric MRI study. *Am J Psychiatr*, **154**, 1424–1429.

Gibbs, M. V., Thorpe, J. G. (1983) Personality stereotype of noninstitutionalized Down Syndrome children. *Am J Ment Defic*, **87**, 601–605.

Gibson, D. (1978) *Down's Syndrome: The Psychology of Mongolism*. Cambridge: Cambridge University Press.

Gunn, P., Berry, P. (1985) Down's syndrome temperament and maternal response to descriptions of child behavior. *Dev Psychol*, **21**, 842–847.

Gunn, P., Berry, P., Andrews, R. J. (1982) Looking behavior of Down syndrome infants. *Am J Ment Defic*, **87**, 344–347.

Gunn, P., Cuskelly, M. (1991) Down syndrome temperament: the stereotype at middle childhood and adolescence. *International Journal of Disability, Development, and Education*, **38**, 59–70.

Heiman, M., Ullstadius, E. (1999) Neonatal imitation and imitation among children with autism and Down's syndrome. In J. Nadel, G. Butterworth (eds) *Imitation in Infancy*. Cambridge: Cambridge University Press, pp. 235–253.

Hesketh, L. J., Chapman, R. S. (1998) Verb use by individuals with Down syndrome. *Am J Ment Retard*, **103**, 288–304.

Jarrold, C., Baddeley, A. D. (1997) Short-term memory for verbal and visuospatial information in Down's syndrome. *Cognit Neuropsychiatry*, **2**, 101–122.

Jarrold, C., Baddeley, A. D., Hewes, A. K. (1999) Genetically dissociated components of working memory: evidence from Down's and Williams syndrome. *Neuropsychologia*, **37**, 637–651.

Jobling, A. (1998) Motor development in school-aged children with Down syndrome: a longitudinal perspective. *International Journal of Disability, Development and Education*, **45**, 283–293.

Kasari, C., Freeman, S. F. N. (2001) Task-related social behavior in children with Down syndrome. *Am J Ment Retard*, **106**, 253–264.

Kasari, C., Freeman, S., Mundy, P., Sigman, M. D. (1995) Attention regulation by children with Down syndrome: coordinated joint attention and social referencing looks. *Am J Ment Retard*, **100**, 128–136.

Kasari, C., Mundy, P., Yirmiya, N., Sigman, M. (1990) Affect and attention in children with Down syndrome. *Am J Ment Retard*, **95**, 55–67.

Klein, B. P., Mervis, C. B. (1999) Contrasting patterns of cognitive abilities of 9- and 10-year-olds with Williams syndrome or Down syndrome. *Dev Neuropsychol*, **16**, 177–196.

Kneips, L. J., Walden, T. A., Baxter, A. (1994) Affective expressions of toddlers with and without Down syndrome in a social referencing context. *Am J Ment Retard*, **99**, 301–312.

Landry, S. H., Chapieski, M. L. (1990) Joint attention and infant toy exploration: effects of Down syndrome and prematurity. *Child Dev*, **60**, 103–118.

Laws, G. (1998) The use of nonword repetition as a test of phonological memory in children with Down syndrome. *Journal of Child Psychology and Psychiatry and Allied Disciplines*, **39**, 1119–1130.

Legerstee, M., Bowman, T. G., Fels, S. (1992) People and objects affect the quality of vocalizations in infants with Down syndrome. *Early Development and Parenting*, **1**, 149–156.

Lewis, M., Alessandri, S. M., Sullivan, M. W. (1990) Violation of expectancy, loss of control, and anger expression in young infants. *Dev Psychol*, **63**, 630–638.

Miller, J. F., Leddy, M. (1999) Verbal fluency, speech intelligibility, and communicative effectiveness. In J. F Miller, M. Leddy, L. A. Leavitt (eds) *Improving the Communication of People with Down Syndrome*. Baltimore: Brookes, pp. 81–91.

Mon-Williams, M., Tresilian, J. R., Bell, V. E., Coppard, V. L., Jobling, A., Carson, R. G. (2001) The preparation of reach to grasp movements in adults with Down syndrome. *Hum Mov Sci*, **20**, 587–602.

Morss, J. R. (1983) Cognitive development in the Down's syndrome infant: slow or different? *British Journal of Educational Psychology*, **53**, 40–47.

Mundy, P., Sigman, M., Kasari, C., Yirmiya, N. (1988) Nonverbal communication skills in Down syndrome children. *Child Dev*, **59**, 235–249.

Ohr, P. S., Fagen, J. W. (1991) Conditioning and long term-memory in three month old infants with Down syndrome. *Am J Ment Retard*, **96**, 151–162.

Ohr, P. S., Fagen, J. W. (1994) Contingency learning in 9-month-old infants with Down syndrome. *Am J Ment Retard*, **99**, 74–84.

Piaget, J. (1952) *The Origins of Intelligence in Children*. New York: Norton.

Pinter, J. D., Eliez, S., Schmitt, J. E., Capone, G. T., Reiss, A. L. (2001) Neuroanatomy of Down's syndrome: a high-resolution MRI study. *Am J Psychiatr*, **158**, 1659–1665.

Pitcairn, T. K., Wishart, J. G. (1994) Reactions of young children with Down's syndrome to an impossible task. *Br J Dev Psychol*, **12**, 485–489.

Pueschel, S. R., Gallagher, P. L., Zartler, A. S., Pezzullo, J. C. (1987) Cognitive and learning profiles in children with Down syndrome. *Res Dev Disabil*, **8**, 21–37.

Rodgers, C. (1987) Maternal support for the Down's syndrome stereotype: the effect of direct experience of the condition. *J Ment Defic Res*, **31**, 217–278.

Rosner, B. A., Hodapp, R. M., Fidler, D. J., Sagun, J., Dykens, E. M. (2004) Social competence in persons with Prader-Willi, Williams, and Down syndromes. *J Appl Res Intellect Disabil*, **17**, 209–217.

Ruskin, E. M., Kasari, C., Mundy, P., Sigman, M. (1994) Attention to people and toys during social and object mastery in children with Down syndrome. *Am J Ment Retard*, **99**, 103–111.

Sigman, M., Ruskin, E. (1999) Continuity and change in the social competence of children with autism, Down syndrome, and developmental delays. *Monogr Soc Res Child Dev*, **64**, 1–114.

Uzgiris, I. C., Hunt, J. M. (1979) *Infant Performance and Experience: New Findings with the Ordinal Scales*. Urbana: University of Illinois.

Vaughn, B. E., Contreras, J., Seifer, R. (1994) Short-term longitudinal study of maternal ratings of temperament in samples of children with Down syndrome and children who are developing normally. *Am J Ment Retard*, **98**, 607–618.

Vaughn, B. E., Goldberg, S., Atkinson, L., Marcovitch, S., MacGregor, D., Seifer, R. (1994) Quality of toddler-mother attachment in children with Down syndrome: limits to interpretation of strange situation behavior. *Child Dev*, **65**, 95–108.

Vlachou, M., Farrell, P. (2000) Object mastery motivation in pre-school children with and without disabilities. *Educ Psychol*, **20**, 167–176.

Walden, T., Knieps, L., Baxter, A. (1991) Contingent provision of social referential info by parents of children with and without developmental delays. *Am J Ment Retard*, **96**, 177–187.

Wang, P. P., Bellugi, U. (1994) Evidence from two genetic syndromes for a dissociation between verbal and visuo-spatial short-term memory. *J Clin Exp Neuropsychol*, **16**, 317–322.

Wetherby, A. M., Yonclas, D. G., Bryan, A. A. (1989) Communicative profiles of preschool children with handicaps: implications for early identification. *Journal of Speech and Hearing Disorders*, **54**, 148–158.

Wishart, J. G. (1996) Avoidant learning styles and cognitive development in young children. In B. Stratford, P. Gunn (eds) *New Approaches to Down Syndrome*. London: Cassell, pp. 157–172.

Wishart, J. G., Bower, T. G. R. (1984) Spatial relations and the object concept: a normative study. In L. P. Lipsitt, C. K. Rovee-Collier (eds) *Advances in Infancy Research*, Vol. 3. Norwood: Ablex, pp. 57–123.

Wishart, J. G., Duffy, L. (1990) Instability of performance on cognitive tests in infants and young children with Down's syndrome. *Brit J Educ Psychol*, **60**, 10–22.

Wishart, J. G., Johnston, F. H. (1990) The effects of experience on attribution of a stereotyped personality to children with Down's syndrome. *J Ment Defic Res*, **34**, 409–420.

10 Learning Difficulties in Down Syndrome

GIOVANNI MARIA GUAZZO

Centro NeapoliSanit, Ottaviano (Napoli), Italy

SUMMARY

This chapter summarises the major learning difficulties experienced by individuals with Down syndrome (DS), Williams syndrome (WS) and fragile-X syndrome (FXS). A systematic comparison of learning difficulties and functioning in these three conditions reveals the existence of partial syndrome specificity. Major theoretical and clinical implications of this are outlined. The second half of the chapter discusses the main stages of instructional intervention in intellectual disabilities with particular reference to DS. A lifespan perspective is proposed for such intervention in cases of DS. This is subdivided into three stages:

- the early identification and frequent monitoring of students experiencing learning difficulties
- the schoolwide establishment of long-term learning goals and intermediate performance benchmarks
- the development of coordinated and differentiated instructional interventions for all learners

It is not sufficient to pay attention to special education students and staff. Planning should involve all stakeholders in researching, discussing and examining the entire educational programme. Real inclusion involves restructuring of a school's entire programme and requires constant assessment of practice and results.

An ideal instructional service for people with mental retardation should be comprehensive, coordinated, effective and efficient, incorporating the principles of normalisation and integration and delivered in ways that preserve the clients' dignity and value as equal citizens. It should possess the multidisciplinary skills required for assessment, diagnosis, treatment, care and rehabilitation. Running such a service will no doubt a great challenge for professional staff. Adequate resources, manpower and training are needed to make it successful.

Down Syndrome: Neurobehavioural Specificity. Edited by JA Rondal and J Perera.
© 2006 John Wiley & Sons Ltd.

INTRODUCTION

The relationship between cognitive operation and the ability to learn is extremely complex. There is no direct correlation between the cognitive organisation found in children and their educational achievement. For many years there has been a debate in the field of mental retardation between the cognitive retardation hypothesis and the disorder hypothesis. The current view is that retardation leads to atypical cognitive processes (Zigler & Hodapp 1986; Detterman 1987). In fact, mental retardation can always produce, in time, a clinical picture characterised by atypical cognitive organisation, which correlates either with the degree of retardation or with the specificity of the competences involved. It is necessary to move from a theory of mental retardation based on lack of intelligence to a theory based on how the intelligence that exists works in order to understand when a child with mental retardation has acquired cognitive structures and how that child uses or fails to use the cognitive structures that are available (Gilger & Kaplan 2001).

Many children with mental retardation have particular difficulty passing through the stages of intellectual development and integrating different cognitive strategies. Some of them underuse their abilities and perform below their potential. All children with mental retardation experience difficulty in coping with situations involving transformation and cognitive conflict and this poses a risk that, with time, atypical cognitive processes could occur. In this context, the relationship between intellectual disorder and learning difficulty may be seen as the main problem in the pathology of mental retardation.

We have indicated that cognitive operation problems involve a learning difficulty, the seriousness of which depends on the degree and type of mental retardation and the specificity of which depends on time and the ways in which the individual learns. Many intellectual disorders and learning difficulties exist, resulting in a lack of homogeneity in cognitive and neuropsychological profiles and in diversity in cases of DS. Beyond the possibility of finding parameters for predicting scholastic difficulties in children with mental retardation and identifying characteristic stages or 'critical moments' in their learning processes, the variability of the clinical pictures in conditions such as DS, WS or FXS should be considered as a point of departure for analysing the relationship between mental retardation and learning difficulty.

MENTAL RETARDATION, LEARNING DIFFICULTIES AND SOME GENETIC SYNDROMES

Mental retardation accounts for the greatest percentage of handicapped people. Estimates range from 80% to 90%. According to the American Association on Mental Retardation (2002) the term 'mental retardation' refers to general intellectual functioning meaningfully inferior to the norm, originating during the period from birth to the age of 18 years. It is associated with problems in adapting to life in two or more of a number of fields including communication, home life, use of community resources and health (Grossman 1977). In other words, mental retardation is a condition in which general intellectual functioning is meaningfully below average (IQ < 70) and is associated with a deficit in adaptive behaviour.

Mental retardation constitutes one of the more important problems in primary school because of the frequency with which it appears and because of the difficulty in differentiating it from other clinical profiles that, despite various aetiologies, have the same symptomatology.

From this point of view, instead of the traditional classification into subgroups (*mild:* IQ 50–70, approximately 80% of cases; *moderate:* IQ 35–49, approximately 12% of cases; *severe:* IQ 20–34, approximately 7% of cases; *most severe:* IQ ≤ 20, approximately 1% of cases) clinicians specialising in mental retardation have preferred to use a model that examines interactions among intelligence disorders, development and learning in more depth (Macmillan et al. 1986). If we want to understand children's cognitive organisation it is essential to know the time when particular cognitive functions emerge in every stage.

However, it is a common view that all cases of moderate, severe or very severe mental retardation have an organic cause. It should therefore be easy to characterise abnormal development of the brain, whether the cause is genetic or not. Among genetic causes DS, WS and FXS have been studied most, especially in recent decades (Table 10.1).

DOWN SYNDROME

The most frequently occurring genetic syndrome is DS, also known as 'trisomy 21'. Its occurrence is currently approximately 1 in every 1000 live births.

Table 10.1. Three profiles of learning difficulties: Down, Williams and fragile-X syndromes. The sign '+' means relative strength and '−' means relative weakness

LEARNING DIFFICULTIES	SYNDROMES		
	Down	Williams	Fragile-X
Language			
• Expressive	−	+	−
• Receptive	−	+	−
• Pragmatic	+	−	−
Reading	−	+	−
Writing	−	+	−
Mathematics	−	+	−
Metacognition	−	+	−

Cases of trisomy 21 are usually classified in three aetiological subcategories:

- standard trisomy 21 (97% of cases)
- mosaicism (1% of cases) and
- translocation (2% of cases)

Down syndrome has been studied most, especially in recent decades. Although much information has been collected about DS, this does not mean that all aspects of the syndrome, its development, pathologies and related problems have been explored. We are often inclined to consider this syndrome as typical of moderate and severe mental retardation. This is dangerous, and probably inaccurate. Comparison with other genetic mental retardation syndromes suggests that it is more variable and has a degree of syndrome specificity.

WILLIAMS SYNDROME

This syndrome involves a rare metabolic disorder and its frequency is approximately 1 birth in every 20000, with a higher incidence in males than in females. The aetiological mechanism responsible for WS is an anomaly in chromosome 7. Individuals with WS have a particular psychological profile. In general, there is:

- a dissociation between language and attitude
- the existence of a severe spatial cognition deficit and
- important problems with movements, especially 'fine' movements

Individuals with WS frequently display a weakness in visual perception: these children and adolescents experience many difficulties in integrating the different parts of a visual whole in a coherent and functional way. This type of problem is evident in their drawings and in other graphical representations. It has been observed, for example, that they are not really able to draw a complex object like a bicycle. Their drawings show a 'dispersion' of different components of the composed object without functional integration. Individuals with DS often draw badly but the object is integrated and it can therefore be recognised easily. Another characteristic of WS is a minor language deficit. Pragmatic (social) use of language – for example, talking correctly and effectively according to the cultural and linguistic rules that exist in the community – is problematic for children and adolescents with WS. There is therefore a contrast between the language problems of individuals with WS and those with DS. The latter more often have big problems with articulation and morphosyntax. However their communicative and pragmatic functioning is more appropriate.

FRAGILE-X SYNDROME

Individuals with FXS show a null mutation of gene FMR-1 (in position q27 of chromosome X) in which the protein levels of DNA (deoxyribosenucleic acid) are substantially reduced. It is difficult to establish the exact incidence of the syndrome because many cases go unidentified. Eighty per cent of male subjects have moderate mental retardation; the others have normal intelligence. About a third of female carriers have a variation of the FXS that includes learning difficulties. Some of these women show a mild mental retardation. The others are normal but they can transmit the genetic problem to their sons.

Individuals with FXS experience difficulty with verbal and visual memory, attention deficit, hyperactivity and a tendency to impulsiveness. Males, in particular, have serious difficulties in controlling speech rhythm is concerned. Vocal problems, dysrhythmia, echolalia and reduced intelligibility of language have also been observed. Language can also be inappropriate at the pragmatic level.

Careful reading of these observations provides many meaningful indications about the cognitive factors involved in learning.

COGNITIVE FACTORS AND THE HUMAN INFORMATION PROCESSING MODEL

Cognitive processes can be defined as representations and mental processes (perception, attention, memory, thought) that allow the individual to perceive and to elaborate information that is essential for behaviour and that allow the individual to know the world. This formulation, which has existed since the 1960s, is central to the *human information processing* (HIP) paradigm, which considers the human being like a computer (Neisser 1967; Atkinson & Shiffrin 1968; Cohen 1983).

As Figure 10.1 shows, information can be processed at various levels and items of information can be processed either sequentially (serial processing) or in parallel (parallel processing) (Neisser 1963; Guazzo 1987, 1991). Moreover, this can happen inside a person (for example, when recalling a past acquaintance) or between the individual and the environment (for example, reading or observing). In the latter case the individual receives information from the external world through the sense organs. Each of these is connected with a sensory register where the information is held for a short period of time (approximately 1 s). These sensory memories are better understood as part of the primary processing system. Both sight and hearing seem to have temporary stores.

This allows sensory information to be integrated with information that comes from other sources. Information held in this way is sent to the long-term memory system, which codes principally in terms of meaning but is also

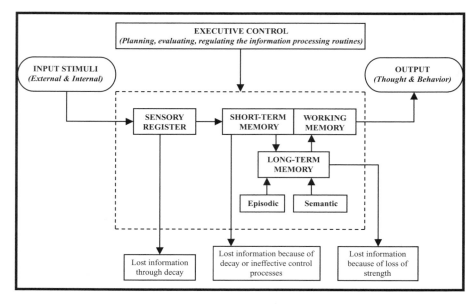

Figure 10.1. The *human information processing* model proposes that information is processed and stored in three stages: 1 sensory register, 2 short-term memory (also called working memory), and 3 long-term memory (this memory is comprised of a number of interrelated subsystems including episodic and semantic memory).

able to store some sensory characteristics like those involved in memory for faces, voices or sounds. The information is subsequently sent to the short-term memory (STM).

In the STM information is held for a slightly longer period (about 10 s). The system only saves a small amount of information at a time. Typically STM carries out roles such as remembering the order in which sequential information has been received to avoid omissions and similar errors (Guazzo 1987). The span of memory is measured by asking a subject to repeat a series of unconnected items. The span has some interesting properties:

• For items in random order the span is seven, plus or minus two. The amount of information in the items has little effect on the span.
• The span is not influenced by the speed with which the elements are introduced and therefore is relatively independent of the time that passes between the presentation of an item and its memorisation.
• The span is reduced if the elements of the sequence have a similar sound. For example, the sequence D P T V is more difficult than the sequence E F H M.
• The span is smaller for long words than for short ones.

These points are explained by so-called *chunk theory*. According to this theory, the span indicates that the brain has the ability to store approximately seven chunks. Every chunk is in a position in which a single item can be stored. Once the store is full, new items can be only be stored by moving existing ones. Variations in the span, according to this theory, can be attributed to the fact that a chunk can sometimes contain more than one item – for example, two or more digits can sometimes be recoded like a number that is familiar, which can be stored as one chunk. Individuals who are familiar with the numbers can have spans of 15 or more units (Miller 1956).

It is important to analyse how this ability is used in cognitive activity. The STM has a function. The term *working memory* refers to those parts of the system of human memory that are used in order to hold information temporarily and to operate on it to execute mental activities. Reading, writing, speaking, hanging a picture and so forth are activities that require us to work on items of information that cannot all be present at a certain moment but they are partially held in the mind thanks to a system of temporary memory. As a result of these considerations, Baddeley (1986) has proposed that working memory comprises a central executive system of control and two subsystems.

The first subsystem, the articulatory loop, according to Baddeley, is responsible for holding oral information. It consists of a passive store and an active articulation process. This simple model can explain various factors that influence the STM, including acoustic similarity and word length. Moreover, the articulatory loop has an important role in learning reading, understanding language and the acquisition of the vocabulary. In such tasks working memory is constantly used to hold information. People who read must remember the information as soon as they have read it in order to process it. People who learn to read must memorise sequences of phonemes in order to combine them. People who write must remember other parts of the text. For example, if someone dictates a sentence with five words, while we are writing the first we must remember all the others. People who make calculations must hold the information about the rules and about operations that they have already performed (Kluwe 1982; Cornoldi 1986; Whittaker 1988; Wood & Terrel 1998).

Baddeley's second subsystem is the visuospatial note-book – a system that controls the preparation and manipulation of visual images, but not for long-term oral memory. It is probably a system with both visual and spatial parts. Many studies (Ungerleider & Mishkin 1982; Weiskrantz 1986) have demonstrated that the visual system consists of two components, one involved in the elaboration of complex stimuli and to identifying what they are (the 'what system') and the other involved in spatial location of the stimuli (the 'where system').

Most of the research on working memory has been concentrated on the two subsidiary systems. The central executive system is the third component.

According to Baddeley its function is to select strategies, to manage the available resources, to integrate the information coming from various sources and to coordinate the execution of various activities when they are carried out at the same time. In a sense, therefore, the central executive works more like an attention system than a memory store and we could therefore start by examining some theories of attention hoping that they can give us a model for working memory (Brown 1975; Daneman & Carpenter 1980; Baddeley 1990).

Most theories of attention that have been proposed are strongly influenced by communication theory and by computer science technology. The existence of a variety of theories is due in some measure to the variety of the phenomena that can be grouped under the label 'attention'. These phenomena include, for example, our ability to listen selectively to one message while ignoring another, to watch a figure in a particular colour in presence of other colours, and to maintain a high level of attention (vigilance).

Although no one theory is dominant, filter theory (Broadbent 1958) continues to exert an influence. Broadbent has proposed that there is a single central channel of information in the brain whose analytical abilities are quite limited. This central channel can select, at a particular time, a single sensory channel for incoming information, and it cannot change from one channel to another more quickly than twice per second. Accepting incoming information in equivalent to paying attention to that source of information, while the information on the channel to which you don't pay attention can be maintained briefly in short-term memory. Broadbent has called the selection mechanism a 'filter'. With practice you can see remarkable improvements in performance, and some authors, among them Kahneman (1973), have proposed a parallel processing model of attention. The main limitation, according to this model, is one's ability to make an effort, rather than competition among separate channels of information. Norman & Shallice (1986) propose a model that provides a general explanation for the way in which action is controlled. This seems to offer a useful basis for conceptualising the executive component of working memory.

Norman and Shallice stated that most actions are controlled by schemata – series of actions that are executed automatically once they have been started correctly. Such schemata can operate at various levels, from responses to the simple touch of a feather on the skin, to walking, to more complex processes like those involved in using a computer or writing a letter. Different schemata can be in operation simultaneously – for example you can walk and speak to a friend at the same time. Both these activities proceed with minimal attention control; attention is concentrated on organising the next concept. If they were not organised, such schemata would probably come into conflict at times, leading to the destruction of the behaviour. In this model the conflict is eliminated by an automatic process that selects one of the conflicting schemata, environmental cues indicating which should be given precedence at a given moment. In addition to this process of resolution of the automatic conflict there is a general controller, the supervisory attention system (SAS) (Figure 10.2). This system has a limited function and Norman and Shallice identify it with the will. It is used in various situations:

- tasks that demand planning or a decision
- situations in which automatic processes seem to have difficulty
- when sequences of new or unfamiliar actions are involved
- when the situation is judged to be difficult

The model assumes that actions are controlled at two levels. First, through the solution of conflicts among schemata. This eliminates the production of incompatible actions and prevents overloading the subcomponents of the system. Second, there is the general supervision of the SAS. The model of Norman and Shallice seems to offer a good explanation of the operation of the central executive of the working memory (Mandler 1967; Schneider & Pressley 1989).

Eventually information passes into long-term memory (LTM). This is relatively permanent in comparison with the STM. Here information is conserved

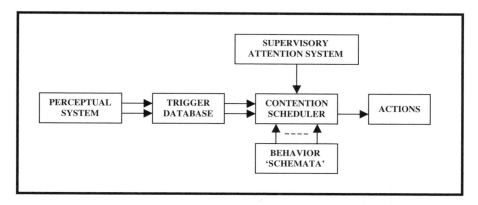

Figure 10.2. The Norman & Shallice (1986) model for willed and automatic control of behaviour. A perceptual subsystem, via an associative database, causes a range of behaviours to be 'triggered' for possible expression. For each behaviour, the strength of the triggering depends upon the applicability of that behaviour to the perceived state of the environment. The associative mapping takes account of the internal state of the agent and any goals that it has. A 'willed' action component is applied by supervisory attention system (SAS) which modulates behaviour selection to correct errors and invoke actions to deal with novelty in the environment. According to Shallice (1988), the SAS is a limited capacity system and is used for a variety of purposes, including: tasks involving planning or decision making, troubleshooting in situations in which the automatic processes appear to be running into difficulty, novel or dangerous or technically difficult situations and situations where strong habitual responses or temptations are involved.

and recovered using a search process. Long-term memory is the store where everything that the individual knows is held: names, experiences, acquaintances and so forth (Guazzo 1987).

Various studies have indicated the presence of cognitive and memory difficulties in mental retardation that can be attributed to strategic deficits. The extent to which these have been noticed varies depending upon the methodology, the type of test, the material used and the type of retardation studied (Ellis 1970; Forness & Kavale 1993; Bower & Hayes 1994; Dobson & Rust 1994). Studies of cognitive aspects of DS have shown particularly inadequate performance in both short-term and long-term memory tasks, compared with other types of mental retardation (Ellis et al. 1989; Ohr 1991). Individuals with DS have difficulties with oral span, in the immediate inverse recall of oral and visual-spatial sequences because of the lack of the recency effect, in the use of the categorical organisation and in the acquisition of language (Varnhagen & Varnhagen 1987; Marcell & Weeks 1988; Forness & Kavale 1993; Bower & Hayes 1994; Fowler et al. 1994; Fletcher & Bray 1995; Marcell et al. 1995; Vicari et al. 1995).

Compared with normal children and with mentally retarded non-Down children, Down children show greater difficulties with auditory-type processes than visual-type processes and therefore, at least at the level of STM, they are worse at remembering stimuli introduced orally than those introduced visually (Marcell & Weeks 1988). Down children could therefore experience some difficulties in understanding instructions pronounced orally or introduced in an oral way and would benefit when they are assisted by a practical demonstration. Mentally retarded non-Down individuals show some memory deficits both in encoding and storing information. Moreover, they behave in an extremely rigid way, especially when the task is too difficult for them – when it demands cognitive resources that exceed those that are available (Kreitler et al. 1990).

Mentally retarded individuals (Down and non-Down) demonstrate greater strategic learning abilities when the strategy is external and perform worse with oral strategies (Bray et al. 1994a, 1994b; Ferretti 1994; Fletcher & Bray 1995). In this respect they are similar to those infants who benefit from external mnemonic aids but have greater difficulties when instructions are orally expressed (De Loache & Todd 1988).

However, many studies indicated that the gap between the various types of mentally retarded individuals and normal ones at physical, social and cognitive levels can be reduced by adapting environmental stimulation, by parental expectations and by the use of appropriate evaluation and rehabilitation techniques (Turner et al. 1994; Buchel 1990; Scruggs & Mastropieri 1993; Rosenthal et al. 1994; Shiffrin & Schneider 1977).

As we have seen, one fundamental characteristic of memory is the use of strategies. A strategy is essentially a method used to reach an objective (Guazzo 1987; Ashman & Conway 1989). It implies a more-or-less controlled attempt to adapt cognitive processes to the requirements of a task in order to reach an objective. Moreover, the strategies are modifiable and can be made more effective. The ability to execute a task can be hindered by three types of problem: limited ability, not knowing how to use the adopted strategy and inefficient use of strategies (Cavanough & Perlmutter 1982; Wellman 1985; Guazzo 2004).

A distinction has been made between production deficiency and mediation deficiency (Flavell 1970, 1971). A production deficiency is assumed if the student does not use a memory strategy spontaneously but can use it if trained; a mediation deficiency exists when the student produces a strategy that does not improve performance. The objective of instruction therefore is to enable students to manage their own learning through the use of strategies.

Attention influences both the storage of information in memory and its recovery. Attention includes all the mechanisms and the processes through which individuals can consciously act on their mental activity, control the external environment, programme plans of action, execute them and estimate the results.

Let us now consider learning from an information-processing standpoint (Flavell 1985).

Learning has a constructive character. Acquired knowledge is constructed, rather than recorded or accepted. Such construction is influenced by the way in which previous knowledge has been structured. The process of assimilating new information and experiences implies the organisation of past reactions and experiences in cognitive structures called *schemas*. The schema is a complex cognitive unit that is neither an image nor a photographic copy of an event but rather the abstract representation of events (Rumelhart & Ortony 1977). The schema of a face for an infant, for example, probably comprises one figure containing two oval circles arranged horizontally (the eyes). Once the schema of a phenomenon has been formed, the infant is inclined to pay attention to those stimuli that are a little different, but not completely, from those that characterise the original schema. A schema has some attributes that can vary in different situations where it is 'adopted' – for example, the face schema does not specify the colour of the eyes or the largeness of the forehead but it specifies the presence of these elements (Norman & Borrow 1975; Norman 1982).

The adoption of the schema as the basic element of knowledge acquisition has two fundamental implications for educational psychology planning. The first implication is the dynamic character of the acquisition of the knowledge, which proceeds through the use, modification and reorganisation of structures that elaborate the experience and are, in turn, influenced by it. The second implication regards the continuity of the newly acquired knowledge with what has been remembered. If knowing always involves the construction of information based on accumulated knowledge acquisition, learning is never repetitive (Guazzo 1987). Some authors (Bransford 1979; Jenkins 1979; Rohwer 1984) have considered learning to be the result of an interaction between the various cognitive processes and between these and metacognitive processes (Flavell 1976, 1979, 1981); that is, they have developed interactive models of learning that analyse the relationships between the following factors:

- characteristics of the students: their specific cognitive and metacognitive abilities, the strategies they have acquired, their cognitive styles, motivations, expectations, and so forth
- the learning activities: the actual cognitive processes (such as attention, understanding, thought) and the strategies used by students in those particular tasks
- the characteristics of the material to be learned: the texts, and the order of exposure to the material, the presence of questions and so forth
- the quality of the instruction: the methodology chosen by the teacher and the teacher's ability to communicate with the students
- the test: whether it consists of a questionnaire, multiple-choice questions, interrogation and so forth – the result of a test is influenced by various factors such as the students' knowledge and their expectations about themselves

LEARNING DIFFICULTIES IN DOWN SYNDROME

The term 'learning difficulties' refers to a heterogeneous group of difficulties that encapsulate a diverse range of problems in cognitive development and scholastic learning. They may be defined in terms of the failure to attain important criteria in particular fields such as reading, writing, calculation and language. They often present at the same time although not necessarily with the same intensity.

READING DIFFICULTIES

Reading difficulties are probably the most well known learning difficulties and have been studied most. A reading difficulty is a specific and meaningful disorder in the development of reading ability that is not explained by mental age, by visual problems or inadequate instruction but by the lexical and phonological strategies used when someone reads. There are various types of error:

- visual errors, which consist of mistaking letters that appear similar (for example, 'e' with 'a', 'm' with 'n', 'b' with 'd')
- phonological errors – for example, in Italian, 'f' with 'v', 'c' with 'g'
- 'anticipation' errors – a word is read in place of another, which is similar either in terms of its initial letters or its meaning

These errors can be identified using tests (Ross 1974; Martin 1971) and theoretical models exist to account for them (Coltheart 1981; Frith 1985). The ability to decode while reading and the ability to understand are substantially independent – a finding that is confirmed in the international literature but appears particularly true for Italians whose phonological regularity allows them to read without understanding what they have read.

WRITING DIFFICULTIES

The term 'writing difficulties' is used in order to describe very heterogeneous clinical pictures in which cognitive or linguistic disorders can reveal themselves either together with other pathologies or in an isolated way. The acquisition of specific competences involves the integration of complex functions (sensomotor, neurocognitive and socioemotional). A failure in the evolution of one or more of these components can have important consequences (Johnson & Myklebust 1967). Writing difficulties are associated more with visuomotor coordination than the development of the language. Difficulties can be revealed by tasks requiring individuals to reproduce a graphical sign from memory or to copy a letter. These problems also seem be related to difficulties in drawing and, more generally, to the apraxias and dispraxias. These praxic disorders cause writing problems either because younger children are incapable of writing letters, or because older children control their writing poorly, resulting in visually messy written products.

Writing ability has been studied frequently and a distinction has been made between a phase in which individuals acquire fundamental phonological rules (probably through successively approximation) and a phase in which they learn irregularities (like the groups ch, gh, gl, gn, sc) and exceptions to rules. Writing ability is not only an issue of memory; it is a complex linguistic process (Frith 1980).

Bereiter & Scardamalia (1982) have demonstrated how writing develops from a process based on characteristics of oral production to a system that works independently and requires the child to manage various cognitive processes (lexical access, grammar, planning, and so forth). Moreover, Johnson (1988) has demonstrated many different writing difficulties ranging from the recovery of information from long-term memory through to the planning of the text, to insufficient rereading and revision, to difficulty in assuming the perspective of potential readers.

MATHEMATICAL DIFFICULTIES

The system of the numbers is accessed through various codes. The most important are the oral alphabetical code (for example, the oral word 'five'), the written alphabetical code (the written word 'five') and the arabic number code (symbol '5'). To these it is necessary to add a pictographic code and the roman system of numbers (which requires the use of alphabetical signs, in this case 'V').

Each time that we change from one code to another it is necessary to use numerical transcoding. Transcoding means producing a number introduced in one code using a different code. Writing arabic numbers that are being dictated constitutes an example of transcoding from the oral alphabetical code to the arabic code. Reading in a loud voice involves transcoding from the arabic code to the oral alphabetical code and so on.

Researchers recognise particular characteristics in the system used for calculation. First, it is functionally dependent on the system of the numbers, which it uses both for processing the numbers and in order to supply the result of the operation. The calculation system, moreover, seems to be structured according to three nonhierarchical levels, which are activated according to the type of arithmetical task required:

- attribution of procedures to algebraic signs – for example, adding if the '+' sign appears, multiplying if '×' appears, and so forth
- 'numerical operations' such as reading tables, simple calculation and other tasks that you can approach without executing an algorithm to produce a solution
- calculation procedures that involve, for example, written calculation, following an algorithm

Children know that they should use a system of procedures and algorithms in order to resolve numerical and arithmetical tasks. In order to do this they use the information and the instructions that they receive from adults or from more expert children. In part they demonstrate their abstraction and generalisation abilities, applying learned knowledge to new tasks.

The difficulties that the children can encounter do not involve all mathematical learning but only some basic numerical and arithmetical tasks, such as numerical processing and calculation.

LANGUAGE DIFFICULTIES

The term 'language difficulties' is used to describe very heterogeneous clinical profiles where linguistic difficulties can manifest themselves in combination with other pathological conditions (neuromotor, sensorial, cognitive and relational deficits) or in isolation.

For an analysis of language difficulties in typical and atypical development and in DS see Rondal's chapter in this volume.

As we have seen, the relationship between cognitive development and scholastic learning is extremely complex and involves the interaction of different functions. In order to understand learning difficulties in children with DS two general premises are necessary:

- basic cognitive disorders limit the amount and the quality of the mental operations possible in every phase of the process of development
- the evolution of mental retardation involves the development of functions and dysfunctions that can integrate in an atypical way, compete or be dissociated

This means that, for DS children, the risk of confusion or inappropriate reactions to new learning is always present.

In DS there is considerable evidence of the complexity of the relationship between cognitive disorder and learning difficulty. The wide variability of the school profiles of the Down children, in terms of the seriousness, the typology and the evolution of learning difficulties, is an indication of the complexity of the problem. Some cognitive and neuropsychological competences correlate with the acquisition of reading and writing and can be used to forecast scholastic outcomes. Among these competences (including the ability to use syllables, words, phrases, oral understanding, written language), competence with the written syllable – the first functional unit of the process of acquisition of reading and writing – and the time at which this competence is acquired is the simplest parameter for analysing the learning process. This analysis shows that only children with very inadequate linguistic competence have great difficulties in the learning process. The very slow acquisition of the first functional unit of written language seems, therefore, in itself, to constitute an element of risk that threatens the child's ability to progress to more complex learning. Moreover, it appears closely correlated with the levels of cognitive and linguistic organisation reached (both in terms of the number of skills acquired and times of acquisition). It is like a 'critical' moment in the process of learning to move between oral and written language.

From a clinical point of view, we have to consider what 'use' children are making of their own skills during the process of acquisition of reading and writing. Such knowledge allows us to plan therapeutic, didactic and social interventions that better target the real requirements of Down children (Capozzi et al. 1991).

GUIDELINES FOR TREATMENT AND INTERVENTION

The most common and most accepted treatment for learning disabilities in DS has been educational intervention. Every treatment and intervention programme starts with a thorough assessment of the child's deficits and assets in the context of a multidisciplinary evaluation including assessments of behavioural history and current presentation, neuropsychological functioning, communication pattern, learning skill and adaptive functioning (Lidz 1990; Buchel 1990). The final formulation should include a characterisation of the child's deficits and abilities in these various areas. Then it is absolutely crucial that the intervention programme derived from this comprehensive evaluation is individualised to insure that it addresses the unique profile of needs and strengths exhibited by the child.

Specific intervention – the practices and approaches, behavioural management techniques, strategies for emotional support, and activities intended to foster scholastic and communication competence – should be conceived and implemented in a thoughtful, consistent (across settings, between parents, between general and special education teachers, rehabilitation therapists, and so forth) and individualised manner. More importantly, the benefit (or lack thereof) of specific recommendations should be assessed in an empirical fashion (based on an evaluation of events observed, documented or charted) with useful strategies being maintained and unhelpful ones discarded so as to promote a constant adjustment of the programme to the specific conditions of the individual child with DS. The following set of guidelines reflects our clinical and research experience in learning disabilities with DS in the past few years. It should not be applied in specific cases without a thoughtful discussion of the individual child's profile. The guidelines should be seen as a series of suggestions to be considered when planning for the individual's educational and treatment (Guazzo 2004):

- There should be an assessment and teaching process with referral stages (prereferral, referral and initial planning), assessment stages (multidisciplinary evaluation, individual educational project meeting) and instruction stages (implementing the teaching plan, monitoring progress).
- Present levels of performance should be noted.
- There should be annual goals and benchmarks (short-term objectives).
- Special education services are needed.
- There should be a projected date for these services to begin as well as details of their frequency, location and duration.
- There should be measures of progress toward annual goals.

CONCLUSIONS

All Down children show a learning disturbance during their development, which manifests itself at different times and in different ways according to the seriousness of retardation and the evolution of the neuropsychological profile. The difficulties that this population experiences in learning to read and write can be viewed in various ways – for example as simple delays or serious deficits. The heterogeneity of this population means that it is necessary to use reliable parameters, such as the times of acquisition of particular development pointers, to help us to make a diagnosis about the extent and seriousness of the delay. We should then analyse the appearance of simple but significant parameters (like the use of syllables) that allow us to make estimates about their learning.

The educational focus will be on the attainment of better logic-linguistic integration. At first treatment will strengthen the relationship between praxic and linguistic competences. When children are able to represent actions, words and feelings, they can begin to learn new codes such as reading and writing.

REFERENCES

American Association on Mental Retardation (2002) *Mental Retardation. Definition, Classification, and Systems of Support*. Washington DC: AAMR.

Ashman, A. F., Conway N. F. (1989) *Cognitive Strategies for Special Education*. New York: Routledge.

Atkinson, J. W., Shiffrin R. M. (1968) Human memory: a proposed system and its control processes. Advances in the research and theory. In K. W. Spence (ed.) *The Psychology of Learning and Motivation*. New York: Academic Press.

Baddeley, A. (1986) *Working Memory*. Oxford: Clarendon Press.

Baddeley, A. (1990) *Human Memory. Theory and Practice*. Hove: Lawrence Erlbaum Associates.

Bereiter, C., Scardamalia, M. (1982) From conservation to composition: the role of instruction in a developmental process. In R. Glaser (ed.) *Advances in Instructional Psychology*, Vol. 2. Hillsdale NJ: Erlbaum.

Bower, A., Hayes, A. (1994) Short-term memory deficits and Down's syndrome: a comparative study. *Down's Syndrome Res Pract*, **2**, 47–50.

Bransford, J. D. (1979) Prerequisites for the utilization of knowledge in the recall of prose passages. *Journal of Experimental Psychology: Human Learning and Memory*, **5**, 253–261.

Bray, N. W., Saarnio, D. A., Borges L. M., Hawk L. W. (1994a) Intellectual and developmental differences in external memory strategies. *Am J Ment Retard*, **99**(1), 19–31.

Bray, N. W., Saarnio, D. A., Borges L. M., Hawk, L. W. (1994b) Context for understanding intellectual and developmental differences in strategy competencies. *Am J Ment Retard*, **99**(1), 44–49.

Broadbent, D. E. (1958) *Perception and Communication*. London: Pergamon Press.

Brown, A. L. (1975) The development of memory: knowing, knowing about knowing, and knowing how to know. In H. W. Reese (ed.) *Advances in Child Development and Behavior*, Vol. 10. New York: Academic Press.

Buchel, F. P. (1990) Analyse des processus d'apprentissage mediatises aupres d'enfants presentant des difficultes d'apprentissage. *Revue de Psychologie Appliquée*, **40**(4), 407–424.

Capozzi, F., Musatti, L., Levi, G. (1991) I disturbi di apprendimento nel ritardo mentale. In C. Cornoldi (ed.) *I disturbi dell'apprendimento*. Bologna: Il Mulino, pp. 169–188.

Cavanough, J. C., Perlmutter, M. (1982) Metamemory. A critical examination. *Child Dev*, 53.

Cohen, G. (1983) *Psychology of Cognitive Processes*. London: Academic Press.

Coltheart, M. (1981) Disorders of reading and their implications for models of normal reading. *Visible Language*, **15**, 245–286.

Cornoldi, C. (1986) *Apprendimento e memoria nell'uomo.* Torino: UTET.

Daneman, M., Carpenter, P. A. (1980) Individual differences in working memory and reading. *Journal of Verbal Learning and Verbal Behavior*, **19**, 450–466.

De Loache, J. S., Brown, A. L. (1985) Intelligent searching by very young children. *Dev Psychol*, **20**, 37–44.

De Loache, J. S., Todd, C. M. (1988) Young children's use of spatial categorization as a mnemonic strategy. *J Exp Child Psychol*, **46**, 1–20.

Detterman, D. (1987) Theoretical notions of intelligence and mental retardation. *Am J Ment Defic*, **92**, 2–11.

Dobson, E., Rust, J. O. (1994) Memory for objects and faces by the mentally retarded and nonretarded. *J Psychol*, **128**(3), 315–322.

Dweck, C. S. (1986) Motivational processes affecting learning. *Am Psychol*, **41**.

Ellis, N. R. (1970) Memory processes in retarded and normals. In N. R. Ellis (ed.) *International Review of Research in Mental Retardation*, Vol. 4. New York: Academic Press.

Ellis, N. R., Woodley-Zanthos, P., Dulaney, C. L. (1989) Memory for spatial location in children, adults, and mentally retarded persons. *American Journal on Mental Retardation*, **93**(5), 521–527.

Ferretti, R. P. (1994) Cognitive, social, and contextual determinants of strategy production: comments on Bray et al. (1994) *American Journal on Mental Retardation*, **99**(1), 32–43.

Flavell, J. H. (1970) Developmental studies of mediated memory. In H. W. Reese, L. P. Lipsitt (eds) *Advances in Child Development and Behaviour.* New York: Academic Press.

Flavell, J. H. (1971) First discussant's comments. What is memory development the development of? *Hum Dev*, **14**, 272–278.

Flavell, J. H. (1976) Metacognitive aspects of problem solving. In L. B. Resnick (ed.) *The Nature of Intelligence.* Hillsdale NJ: Erlbaum.

Flavell, J. H. (1979) Metacognition and cognition monitoring: a new area of psychological inquiry. *Am Psychol*, **34**, 906–911.

Flavell, J. H. (1981) Cognitive monitoring. In W. P. Dickson (ed.) *Children's Oral Communication Skills.* New York: Academic Press.

Flavell, J. H. (1985) *Cognitive Development.* Englewood Cliffs NJ: Prentice-Hall.

Fletcher, K. L., Bray, N. W. (1995) External and verbal strategies in children with and without mild mental retardation. *Am J Ment Retard*, **99**(4), 363–375.

Forness, S. R., Kavale, K. A. (1993) Strategies to improve basic learning and memory deficits in mental retardation: a meta-analysis of experimental studies. *Education and Strategy Acquisition in Mental Retardation*, **28**(2), 99–110.

Fowler, A. E., Gelman, R., Gleitman, L. R. (1994) The course of language learning in children with Down syndrome. In H. T. Flusberg (ed.) *Constraints on Language Acquisition: Studies of Atypical Children.* Hillsdale NJ: Lawrence Erlbaum Associates Inc, pp. 91–140.

Frith, U. (1980) (ed.) *Cognitive Processes in Spelling.* New York: Academic Press.

Frith, U. (1985) The usefulness of the concept of unexpected reading failure: comments on 'Reading retardation revisited'. *Br J Dev Psychol*, **3**, 15–17.

Gilger, J., Kaplan, B. (2001) A typical brain development: a conceptual schemawork for understanding developmental learning disabilities. *Dev Neuropsychol*, **20**(2), 465–481.

Grossman, H. L. (1977) *Manual on Terminology and Classification in Mental Retardation*. Washington DC, American Association on Mental Deficiency.

Guazzo, G. M. (1987) Spontaneous formation of regions with different properties in neural nets. *Biosystems*, **20**, 237–241.

Guazzo, G. M. (1990) *Psicologia dell'handicap*. Salerno: Ripostes.

Guazzo, G. M. (1991) A formalization of Neisser's model. In T. Kohonen, K. Makisara, O. Simula (eds) *Artificial Neural Networks*. Amsterdam: North Holland, pp. 1423–1426.

Guazzo, G. M. (2004) Fattori cognitivi, emotivi e motivazionali nei disturbi dell'apprendimento. In G. M. Guazzo (ed.) *Disturbi dell'apprendimento e stato emotivo*. Nola NA: IRFID, pp. 7–33.

Jenkins, J. R. (1979) Evaluating error-correction procedures for oral reading. *J Spec Educ*, **13**, 145–156.

Johnson, D. J. (1988) Review of research on specific reading, writing, and mathematics disorders. In J. F. Kavanagh T. J. Truss (eds) *Learning Disabilities*. Parkton MD: York Press, pp. 79–163.

Johnson, D. J., Myklebust, H. (1967) *Learning Disabilities: Educational Principles and Practices*. New York: Grune & Stratton.

Kahneman, D. (1973) *Attention and Effort*. Englewood Cliffs NJ: Prentice Hall.

Kluwe, R. H. (1982) Cognitive knowledge and executive control: metacognition. In D. Griffin (ed.) *Animal Mind – Human Mind*. New York: Springer-Verlag.

Kreitler, S., Zigler, E., Kreitler, H. (1990) Rigidity in mentally retarded and nonretarded children. *Am J Ment Retard*, **94**(5), 550–562.

Lidz, C. S. (1990) The pre-school learning assessment device: an approach to the dynamic assessment of young children. Special issue: assessments of learning and development potential: theory and practices. *Eur J Psychol Educ*, **5**(2), 167–175.

Macmillan, D. L., Keogh, B. K., Jones, R. L. (1986) Special educational research on mildly handicapped learners. In M. C. Wittrock (ed.) *Handbook of Research on Teaching*. New York: Macmillan.

Mandler, G. (1967) Organisation in memory. In K. W. Spence (ed.) *The Psychology of Learning and Motivation*, Vol. 1. New York: Academic Press, pp. 327–372.

Marcell, M. M., Ridgeway, M. M., Sewell, D. H., Whelan, M. L. (1995) Sentence imitation by adolescents and young adults with Down's syndrome and other intellectual disabilities. *J Intellect Disabil Res*, **39**(3), 215–232.

Marcell, M. M., Weeks, S. L. (1988) Short-term memory difficulties and Down's syndrome. *J Ment Defic Res*, **32**, 153–162.

Martin, H. P. (1971) Vision and its role in reading disability and dyslexia. *The Journal of School Health*, **41**, 468–472.

Miller, G. A. (1956) The magical number seven, plus or minus two: some limits on our capacity for processing information. *Psychol Rev*, **63**, 81–97.

Neisser, U. (1963) The multiplicity of thought. In P. C. Wason, P. N. Johnson-Laird (eds) *Thinking and Reasoning*. Harmondsworth: Penguin Books.

Neisser, U. (1967) *Cognitive Psychology*. New York: Appleton-Century-Crofts.

Norman, D. A. (1982) *Learning and Memory*. San Francisco CA: Freeman.

Norman, D. A., Borrow, D. G. (1975) On data-limited and resource-limited processes. *Cognit Psychol*, **7**, 44–64.

Norman, D. A., Shallice, T. (1986) Attention to action: willed and automatic control of behavior. In R. J. Davidson, G. E. Schwarts, D. Shapiro (eds) *Consciousness and*

Self-regulation. Advances in Research and Theory. New York: Plenum Press, Vol. 4, pp. 1–18.

Ohr, P. S. (1991) Learning and memory in Down syndrome infants. *Dissertation Abstract International,* **51**(10-B), 505.

Rohwer, W. D. (1984) An invitation to an educational psychology of studying. *Educ Psychol,* **19**, 1–14.

Rosenthal, M., Andrea, L., Yoshida, R. K. (1994) The effects of metacognitive strategy training on the acquisition and generalization of social skills. *Educ Train Ment Retard Dev Disabil,* **29**(3), 213–221.

Ross, A. O. (1974) *Psychological Aspects of Learning Disabilities and Reading Disorders.* New York: McGraw-Hill.

Rumelhart, D. E., Ortony, A. (1977) The representation of knowledge in memory. In R. C. Anderson, R. J. Spiro, W. E. Montague (eds) *Schooling and the Acquisition of Knowledge.* Hillsdale NJ: Erlbaum.

Schneider, W., Pressley, M. (1989) *Memory Development between 2 and 20.* New York: Springer-Verlag.

Scruggs, T. E., Mastropieri, M. A. (1993) Special education for the twenty-first century: integrating learning strategies and thinking skills. *J Learn Disabil,* **26**(6), 392–398.

Shallice, T. (1988) *From Neuropsychology to Mental Structure.* Cambridge: Cambridge University Press.

Shiffrin, R. M., Schneider, W. (1977) Controlled and automatic human information processing II: perceptual learning, automatic attending and a general theory. *Psychol Rev,* **84**, 155–171.

Turner, L. A., Dofny, E. M., Dutka, S. (1994) Effect of strategy and attribution training on strategy maintenance and transfer. *Am J Ment Retard,* **98**(4), 445–454.

Turner, L. A., Matherne, J. L., Heller, S. S. (1994) The effects of performance feedback on memory strategy use and recall accuracy in students with and without mild mental retardation. *J Exp Educ,* **62**(4), 303–315.

Ungerleider, L. G., Mishkin, M. (1982) Two cortical visual systems. In D. J. Ingle, M. A. Goodale, R. J. W. Mansfield (eds) *Analysis of Visual Behavior.* Cambridge MA: MIT Press.

Varnhagen, C. K., Varnhagen, S. (1987) Auditory and visual memory span: cognitive processing by TMR individuals with Down syndrome or other etiologies. *Am J Ment Defic,* **91**, 398–405.

Vicari, S., Carlesimo, G. A., Caltagirone, C. (1995) Short-term memory in persons with intellectual disabilities and Down syndrome. *J Intellect Disabil Res,* **39**, 532–537.

Weiner, B., Frieze, I., Kukla, A., Reed, L., Rest, S., & Rosenbaum, R. (1971) *Perceiving the Causes of Success and Failure.* Morristown NJ: General Learning Press.

Weiner, B. (1990) History of motivational research in education. *J Educ Psychol,* **82**(4), 616–622.

Weiskrantz, L. (1986) *Blindsight, A Case Study and Implications.* Oxford, Oxford University Press.

Wellman, H. M. (1985) The origins of metacognition. In D. L. Forrest-Pressley, G. E. MacKinnon, T. G. Waller (eds) *Metacognition, Cognition and Human Performance.* New York, Academic Press.

Whittaker, S. J. (1988) Success and maintenance of memory strategies by preschoolers. *Int J Behav Dev*, **11**(3), 345–358.

Wood, C., Terrell, C. (1998) Pre-school phonological awareness and subsequent literacy development. *Educ Psychol*, **18**(3), 253.

Zigler E. F., Hodapp R. M. (1986) *Understanding Mental Retardation*. Cambridge: Cambridge University Press.

11 Off to a Good Start: Early Intervention for Infants and Young Children with Down Syndrome and their Families

DONNA SPIKER

Center for Education and Human Services, SRI International, Menlo Park (California), USA

SUMMARY

Early intervention consists of a range of services for infants, toddlers and preschoolers with disabilities, developmental delays – or who are at risk of delays – and their families (Guralnick 2005). These services range from special instruction for the child to therapies (for example, physical, occupational, speech), family training and a variety of specialised services such as audiology, vision or assistive technology services, diagnosis and evaluation (Spiker & Hebbeler 1999). For children with Down syndrome, the goals of early intervention should be to lay the foundation for the child's lifelong learning so that the child will achieve the highest levels of functioning possible, participate fully in family, school, and community life and have the best quality of life possible (Spiker & Hopmann 1997; Guralnick 2005; Spiker et al. 2005). For the child's family, early intervention lays the foundation for the family to be able to help the child achieve those goals (Bailey et al. 1998).

This chapter discusses early intervention for infants, toddlers and preschoolers with Down syndrome, with reference to specificity. It considers whether there are typical, specific, unique characteristics of infants and young children with Down syndrome that are important for how early intervention programmes serve this population of children and their families.

INTRODUCTION

A child's first five years lay the foundation for entrance into formal schooling, so this chapter will be organised around the five domains of children's school

Down Syndrome: Neurobehavioural Specificity. Edited by JA Rondal and J Perera.
© 2006 John Wiley & Sons Ltd.

identified by the US National Education Goals Panel (NEGP

- ̵ ̵ ̵ ̵ ̵ ̵ ̵ and physical development
- cognition and general knowledge
- communicative skills
- emotional wellbeing and social competence
- approaches to learning

The concept of school readiness applies to all children and includes a broad range of interrelated skills and abilities that affect a child's ability to learn and to be successful in school. Early intervention services should aim to provide the necessary support and services needed to promote the health, development, and wellbeing of the children and the ability of parents and caregivers to support and nurture them.

Efficacy research indicates that early intervention services have many benefits. They can:

- accelerate skill acquisition
- prevent abnormal patterns or functioning
- promote optimal parent-child interactions by providing information and modelling stimulating activities
- provide helpful parent support
- encourage children's participation in inclusive settings (Cunningham 1997; Spiker & Hopmann 1997; Bailey et al. 1998; Gibson & Harris 1988; Guralnick 1997, 2001; Spiker et al. 2005)

COMMENTS ABOUT SPECIFICITY AND EARLY INTERVENTION

There is currently no early intervention that is intended specifically for infants and young children with Down syndrome. Furthermore, there is considerable variability among children with Down syndrome with regard to their rate of skill acquisition, health status and conditions, social, behavioural and temperamental characteristics and developmental and educational outcomes. The issue of specificity with regard to early intervention with infants and young children with Down syndrome concerns the way in which the health and developmental characteristics of these children require special attention. Specific characteristics may suggest certain adaptations in the ways that services are provided. They may also give guidance about the most effective ways that parents and providers can interact with the children in order to promote their optimal development and wellbeing.

When parents and providers are well informed and knowledgeable about characteristics that may be more prevalent in this population they should be more likely to provide the kinds of stimulation, support, and care that will lead to better health and development. For each of the five NEGP domains of school readiness, some of the unique considerations about young children with Down syndrome and their implications for early intervention will be described. Table 11.1 provides a summary of the specificity issues discussed in this chapter. Table 11.2 gives some examples, described in each section, showing possible pathways by which specific child characteristics can influence development and learning. Each section also includes implications for early intervention practice.

HEALTH AND PHYSICAL DEVELOPMENT AND EARLY INTERVENTION

This domain of school readiness includes chronic and acute health conditions, the child's physical growth, gross and fine motor skills, oral-motor skills and sensory capacities. As with all infants and young children, children with Down syndrome need to have access to adequate healthcare, including a regular medical home and a consistent healthcare provider who can become acquainted with the unique health needs of the individual child, treat the child appropriately and educate and assist the family about keeping the child healthy.

There are a number of health issues for children with Down syndrome that need special attention (see Pueschel & Pueschel 1992; Cohen 1999; Roizen 2003). Early in infancy, monitoring for the presence of congenital heart conditions is essential so that infants receive appropriate treatment and management. Audiological problems – including ear, nose, and throat (ENT) problems – and ophthalmologic problems need to be diagnosed early and treated. Many young children with Down syndrome have conditions such as hearing loss, nasal and oral obstructions, oral hypotonia, strabismus and vision loss that can affect early learning, language acquisition, sleep patterns, behaviour, and social interaction patterns, to name a few. Furthermore, there are some data to suggest that children with Down syndrome may have a higher incidence of a number of other health conditions that can affect their early development and functioning. These include generalised hypotonia and joint laxity, sleep disorders and difficulties, gastrointestinal disorders such as coeliac disease, obesity and periodontal disease (VanDyke 1995). It is therefore clear that monitoring and addressing the health and physical development issues of young children with Down syndrome is critical. Medical care must monitor physical health and growth, including fine and gross motor development, nutrition and feeding issues, sleep, and sensory functioning. Physical and occupational therapies can also address these needs (Winders 1997; Bruni 1998; Kumin et al. 2001).

Table 11.1. Summary of Down syndrome specificity issues: domains of children's school readiness and early intervention

1. Physical wellbeing and motor development

Children may have difficulties with:
- Congenital heart disorders.
- Audiological and ear, nose, and throat (ENT) disorders:
  - Hearing loss.
  - Nasal/oral obstructions.
  - Oral hypotonia.
- Ophthalmologic problems:
  - Strabismus.
  - Vision loss.
- Hypotonia and joint laxity.
- Sleep disorders.
- Gastrointestinal disorders (e.g., coeliac disease).
- Obesity.
- Periodontal disease.

Early intervention can help by:
- Monitoring and making referrals for appropriate health and dental care.
- Referring for frequent screening of hearing and vision.
- Providing appropriate physical and occupational therapy.
- Evaluating sleep disorders.
- Educating parents and providers about the special health conditions that may be common in children with Down syndrome.
- Including movement and exercise in intervention activities.

2. Cognition and general knowledge

Children may have difficulties with:
- Auditory short-term memory that can be less well developed that visual short-term memory.
- Sustaining exploration and problem solving (less persistent and goal-directed).
- Short-term memory.

Early intervention can help by:
- Using strategies and materials that have emphasis on visual stimuli:[1]
  - Visual cues.
  - Activity schedules that have pictures and photos.
  - Color-coded picture.
  - Real objects, materials, and actual labels.
  - Sign language and gestures with oral language.
- Including repetition and practice of new and emerging skills.

3. Communicative skills

Children may have difficulties with:

• Prelinguistic communication skills related to:[2]
  • Looking.
  • Smiling.
  • Vocalising.
  • Social interaction.
  • Joint attention.
  • Early vocabulary.
• Expressive language (phonology, syntax, pragmatics) relative to receptive language skills.[3]

Early intervention can help by:

• Using a variety of child-centered activities (e.g., toy play, motor games) to promote child interest and initiative.[4]
• Using all the natural contexts as opportunities for increasing the amount of communication opportunities.[5]
• Using interactions that foster imitation, including multiple visual cues.
• Using signs and gestures and communication boards in conjunction with oral language.[6]
• Helping parents increase the child's vocabulary by:
  • Targeting words related to current phonetic repertoire.
  • Following the child's lead of topic and activity.

4. Emotional wellbeing and social emotional development

Children may have difficulties with:[7]

• Emotional expressiveness, with briefer and less intense expressions.
• Taking the initiative in social interactions.
• Maintaining sustained reciprocal social interactions.
• Being less predictable in social interactions.
• Being less persistent and goal-directed in social interactions.

Early intervention can help by:

• Providing parents with information about child temperament and its possible effects on social interactions.[8]
• Providing parents with information about the ways to interact in responsive ways, including:[9]
  • Using teaching routines that imitate child's vocal acts (continue to take another vocal turn).
  • Using teaching routines that interrupt child's established pattern and then wait for child to take a turn.

Table 11.1. *Continued.*

5. Positive approaches to learning

Children may have difficulties with:	Early intervention can help by:
• Being persistent and goal-directed in problem solving and exploration situations.[10] • Using avoidance strategies in learning contexts or be less open to try new tasks. • Using social ploys to avoid 'hard' tasks.[11]	• Determining activities that sustain the child's engagement and interest and using those to increase participation in learning situations. • Including practice with well-developed skills the child has already mastered. • Using errorless teaching techniques. • Reinforcing the child's attention with tasks using the child's interests. • Pacing tasks with work and breaks.[12]

[1] Hodapp et al. (2003).
[2] Ramruttun & Jenkins (1998).
[3] Chapman (1995).
[4] McCathern et al. (1995).
[5] Roper & Dunst (2003).
[6] Foreman & Crews (1998).
[7] Spiker et al. (2002).
[8] Hepburn (2003).
[9] Warren (2000); Yoder & Warren (2004); Mahoney & Perales (2005).
[10] Wishart (1996, 2001).
[11] Wishart (1996, 2001); Fidler (this volume).
[12] Hepburn (2003).

Table 11.2. Specificity and Down syndrome: possible pathways involving domains of children's school readiness

Dimensions of school readiness	Specificity examples
Health and physical development • Chronic health conditions	1 Congenital heart disorder → Reduced exploration; increased parental anxiety → Fewer and less-stimulating interactions → Delayed acquisition of skills and reduced consolidation of learning.
• Musculoskeletal conditions	2 Hypotonia and reduced arousal → Reduced attention and exploration → Delayed acquisition of skills and reduced consolidation of learning.
• Arousal/activity level	3 Low arousal and activity level → Include exercise and physical movement in learning contexts → Increases arousal and attention to learning and social situations.
• Ear, nose, and throat (ENT) difficulties • Sleep difficulties (e.g, apnea, restless sleep)	4 ENT abnormalities → Sleep apnea → Restless sleep → Increased daytime behavior problems (inattention, irritability) and increased fatigue → Reduced consolidation of learning.
Cognition and general knowledge • Exploration and learning	5 Reduced sustained exploration → Reduced consolidation of learning → Longer amount of time to learn → Slower rate of development → Difficulty in generalising skills and learning.
Communicative development • Visual processing better than auditory processing	6 Language input → Child does not understand verbal input → Decreased attention and comprehension → Poor consolidation of verbal learning
• Social signalling better than auditory processing	7 Language input → Use added visual stimuli, (e.g., signs, toys) → Increased attention and comprehension → Better consolidation of verbal learning
	8 Language input → Child signals comprehension by looking and smiling → But child does not comprehend → Receptive language lags
Emotional wellbeing and social competence • Parent-child interactions • Interactions with peers	9 Hypotonia and low arousability → Muted social responses → Less readable or rewarding cues → Reduced parental responsiveness → Fewer and less stimulating parent-child interactions
Approaches to learning • Mastery motivation • Goal-directedness	10 Working on a difficult task → Disengage from task and smiles at adult or seeks help → Reduced engagement in problem solving → Reduced learning and consolidation of learning

These many health issues are interrelated and can set the stage for developmental difficulties and delays. They can affect early development and the transactional processes that affect it (Spiker & Hopmann 1997; Moore et al. 2002). Early intervention can help parents learn about the possible medical needs of their infants and young children, assist them in treating these conditions, and provide emotional support as needed if significant health impairments are detected.

Early intervention providers can also educate parents about how health issues can affect the child's early learning and their own interactions with the child. Table 11.2 shows four different examples of how health conditions could impact on learning and development. In example 1 a chronic health condition such as a congenital heart disorder may lead to fatigue that may reduce the child's exploration of the environment and may also produce increased parental anxiety about the child. In turn, there may then be fewer and less stimulating interactions as a result of either less child exploration or increases in parental protectiveness, with the result that the child's skill acquisition may be delayed and consolidation of learning may be reduced due to less practice of skills. In example 2, a similar pathway is shown for how hypotonia and reduced arousal can lead to delays in development and reduced consolidation of learning. Example 3 shows a pathway demonstrating how early intervention can be adapted to the child's specific characteristics. In this case, including exercise and physical movement as part of the learning context can serve to counteract the tendency of low arousal and activity level and thereby help the child to be more alert and attentive in learning and social situations.

Finally, in example 4, the pathway shows how specific ENT abnormalities (for example, of the tongue, palate, airway obstructions and oral hypotonia) can contribute to sleep apnea and restless sleep (Stores 1993). These sleep difficulties can in turn lead to increased daytime behavioural problems such as inattention and irritability, as well as fatigue. One intriguing idea that needs to be systematically investigated is how these sleep disturbances can affect early learning. That is, sleep disturbances may lead to reduced consolidation of learning. For this reason, it is essential that the underlying reasons for sleep problems in young children with Down syndrome are identified and treated.

COGNITION, GENERAL KNOWLEDGE AND EARLY INTERVENTION

As shown in example 5 in Table 11.2, this domain of school readiness includes thinking and problem-solving skills, exploration of the environment, the ability to acquire knowledge, information, and ideas and early literacy skills. It is well established that cognitive and intellectual development is a significant lifelong difficulty for children with Down syndrome (see the other chapters in this volume for further discussion). The child's ability to acquire, consolidate and use information and knowledge begins to show delays and deficits early in life (for example, early cause-effect knowledge). These delays and deficits, along with the significant challenges in acquiring and using language, severely limit the child's future academic achievement (Boudreau 2002).

Nevertheless, early intervention has increasingly sought to use the best research-based information available to help young children with Down syndrome acquire cognitive and early literacy skills. This support of critical preliteracy skills sets the stage for later learning so that the child can, for instance, learn to read and succeed academically (Byrne et al. 2002). Many of the specific adaptations needed to support early learning are described in the next two sections.

COMMUNICATIVE SKILLS AND EARLY INTERVENTION

This domain of school readiness includes prelinguistic communication skills, receptive language skills and the phonology, syntax and pragmatics of expressive language skills. Children with Down syndrome have significant delays and deficits in acquiring and using both spoken and written language (Chapman 1995; Chapman et al. 1998). This domain, of course, is intricately related to the social skills domain because children's development of language and communication skills is inherently a social-interactional process. In the early prelinguistic phase of development, research has shown a variety of difficulties in how infants and young children with Down syndrome develop and use skills such as looking, smiling, and vocalising in joint attention interactions, with lower rates of initiating communication and subsequent delays in lexical and grammatical development (Chapman 1995; Caselli et al. 1998; Ramruttun & Jenkins 1998).

Early communication intervention should have the goal of increasing vocalisations, gestures, vocabulary and gaze between objects and adults with whom the child interacts. To take into account tendencies toward a more passive interaction style (described in the next section) social interactions should aim to include a variety of child-centred activities (for example, toy play and motor games) to promote child interest and initiative. Furthermore, it is essential that parents and early interventionists working with the child use all natural situations as opportunities for increasing the amount of communication interactions (Roper & Dunst 2003). To take advantage of the visual processing strength relative to auditory processing, it should be beneficial to engage in interactions that foster imitation, including using multiple visual cues and using signs and gestures and communication boards in conjunction with oral language (Foreman & Crews 1998; Clibbens 2001; Clibbens et al. 2002). Several strategies can also be used to help parents and interventionists increase the child's vocabulary, including targeting words related to the child's current phonetic repertoire and following the child's lead in terms of topic and activity (Girolametto et al. 1998).

These suggestions are based on a large body of research about responsive interactions and intervention approaches. This literature has shown that the amount and quality of language input affects the rate and consolidation of early language skills and that young children who are passive or unresponsive in a variety of ways tend to experience less language input from the adults around them and qualitatively different input (for example more directives, less diverse vocabulary) (Warren 2000; Yoder & Warren 2004). Recent work by Mahoney and his colleagues (Mahoney & Perales 2003, 2005; Kim & Mahoney 2004) demonstrates how a relationship-focused intervention approach with young children with disabilities (including those with Down syndrome) – based on research about early language and communication development and using principles of responsive teaching – can lead to significant improvements in young children's cognitive and language development. The goal of this approach is to encourage parents and providers to use social interaction strategies that are responsive to the child's interests and immediate ongoing behaviour.

Early intervention can help parents and early interventionists understand how language input and social communicative interactions provide the context for children's language and communication development. Knowing that young children with Down syndrome have significant auditory processing difficulties, have relatively better developed visual processing and social signalling skills and may have trouble sustaining social interactions can have implications for early intervention strategies that will be most effective.

These difficulties are illustrated in the examples in Table 11.2. Example 6 shows that if there is language input that the child does not understand, the child may then show decreased attention and comprehension, which ultimately results in poor consolidation of verbal learning. Example 7 suggests that language input that is accompanied by visual stimuli, such as signs or toy and real objects, can lead to increased attention and subsequent comprehension, which ultimately results in better consolidation of learning. Finally, in example 8, after the language input, the child may signal the he or she understands by looking and smiling at the adult but the child may not really comprehend what has been said. As a result, the child's receptive language would not have been developed as a result of this kind of social interaction. Understanding this social interaction pattern can lead adults interacting with young children with Down syndrome to check for comprehension during interactions (for example, including requests or questions for which a motor or other response can verify comprehension).

As will be described in the next section, recent research has shown how responsive teaching models can encourage adult-child interactions that lead to better language and communication development (for example McCathern et al. 1995; Yoder & Warren 2004). Briefly, this model encourages the use of follow-in directives by the adult. These are behavioural or verbal responses related to the child's ongoing behaviour. This leads to the child maintaining joint attention in the social interaction. If the adult then provides verbal input that is directly related to what the child is attending to, the child is much more likely to process the input and thereby learn (improved receptive and expressive language skills). Repeated interactions such as this have been shown to support the early language learning of young children with Down syndrome (Yoder & Warren 2004). Furthermore, this approach helps parents learn how most everyday situations are opportunities for language input and learning, thereby making early intervention something that happens during the child's entire waking day (Roper & Dunst 2003).

EMOTIONAL WELLBEING AND SOCIAL COMPETENCE AND EARLY INTERVENTION

This domain of school readiness relates to children's skills in interacting with adults and peers, including the ability to understand social rules, express empathy, play with peers and develop friendships, as well as emotional expressiveness, security, attachment and self-concept. Studies of infants and young children with Down syndrome have shown them to have certain emotional expressiveness, temperamental and social-interaction qualities or tendencies that can negatively affect their early learning. For instance, their early emotional expressiveness may be more muted, with briefer and less intense emotional expressions (Spiker et al. 2002; Hepburn 2003). They may also show difficulties in social interaction by less frequently taking the initiative in social interactions or maintaining sustained reciprocal social interactions, as well as by being less predictable in reciprocal social interactions (Sigman et al. 1999; Spiker et al. 2002). As will also be described below (in the 'approaches to learning' section), young children with Down syndrome may also have a tendency to be less persistent and goal-directed in learning situations (Wishart 1996, 2001). Early learning often takes place in social interactions with adults, so these social, behavioural, temperamental and learning-style characteristics can confound efforts of parents and early intervention providers to help the children learn and practise new or emerging skills.

In Table 11.2, example 9 illustrates how social interactions can be affected by particular social responsiveness of young children with Down syndrome (see Ratekin 1996; Spiker et al. 2002). For instance, if the infant or young child has hypotonia and/or low arousability, this can lead to muted social responses. These, in turn, can lead to less readable or rewarding cues for the parent or adult who is interacting with the child and thus reduced parental responsiveness (for example, an adult may become more directive, which may not always be responsive to the child's ongoing behaviours and interests). The ultimate result of these patterns may be fewer and less stimulating parent-child interactions needed for the child's optimal development, particularly for language and cognitive development.

APPROACHES TO LEARNING AND EARLY INTERVENTION

This domain of school readiness includes children's behaviours related to task persistence and initiative, mastery motivation, goal-directedness, curiosity, creativity and imagination. Studies with young children with Down syndrome have documented tendencies to be less persistent and goal-directed in problem-solving and exploration situations, to use avoidance strategies in learning contexts or be less open to trying new tasks and to use social ploys to avoid 'hard' tasks (for example, frequent off-task behaviour combined with social smiling and looking) (Wishart 1993, 1999, 2001; Linn et al. 2000; Fidler, this volume). This less-than-optimal learning style or reduced mastery motivation, described as a lower motivation to explore or to be goal directed (Niccols et al. 2003) may be due to lower expectations for mastery and sustained engagement in problem solving from adults, more failure experiences, which contribute to avoidance of challenging tasks and/or less frequent reinforcement for independent efforts (Glenn et al. 2001). This reduced goal directedness can also affect how adults interact with the child, making it harder for them to keep the child engaged for sustained periods of time in learning situations (Landry et al. 1998).

In Table 11.2, example 10 illustrates this counterproductive learning style of many young children with Down syndrome. The child is working on a difficult task but soon the child disengages from the task and smiles at the adult or seeks help. This overuse of social and emotional expressiveness occurs along with the child's reduced engagement in problem-solving situations, which in turn may lead to reduced learning and consolidation of learning. Early interventionists need to be aware of this style, help parents understand it, and develop strategies to minimise its effects of the child's early learning (see Fidler, this volume).

Hepburn (2003) has suggested a number of specific strategies that can be used in interactions and learning situations with young children with Down syndrome to limit this counterproductive learning style and to encourage a more active goal-directed learning style. These include:

- determining activities that sustain the child's engagement and interest and using those to increase learning
- practising with well-developed skills that the child has already mastered
- using errorless teaching techniques

- reinforcing the child's attention when engaged in tasks that interest the child
- pacing tasks with work and breaks

It is noteworthy that many of these suggestions are congruent with the recommendations that emerge from research about responsive teaching and strategies to promote early language and communication skills, as described above.

CONCLUSION

Although early intervention is not specific and unique for children with Down syndrome, an understanding of some of the particular tendencies of infants and young children with Down syndrome can suggest activities and strategies that may be particularly effective for this population. Parents probably assume that there are some unique characteristics associated with Down syndrome that they need to be aware of in order to care for their children and promote their optimal health and development. To some extent, they are correct. However, it is also crucial that parents and early interventionists become familiar with the broader field of early intervention (see Guralnick 2005) as many of the non-specific and intentional strategies that have been developed with all young children with disabilities and delays can work well for young children with Down syndrome. For instance, participation in inclusive settings with typically developing peers is an essential component of preschool programming for young children with Down syndrome (Guralnick 2001). Finally, parents must be full partners in the early intervention and education process (Bailey et al. 1998; VanHooste & Maes 2003). If the parents' needs for accurate information, sensitive emotional support, and access to the latest evidence-based intervention strategies are met (Barnett et al. 2003) they will have the best help and support that we can offer so that they can support their child's health and development and lay the foundation for their child's lifelong learning and quality of life.

REFERENCES

Bailey, D. B., Jr., McWilliam, R. A., Darkes, L. A., Hebbeler, K., Simeonsson, R. J., Spiker, D., et al. (1998) Family outcomes in early intervention: A framework for program evaluation and efficacy research. *Exceptional Children*, **64**, 313–328.

Barnett, D., Clements, M., Kaplan-Estrin, M., Fialka, J. (2003) Building new dreams: Supporting parents' adaptation to their child with special needs. *Infants and Young Children*, **3**, 184–200.

Boudreau, D. (2002) Literacy skills in children and adolescents with Down syndrome. *Read Writ*, **15**, 497–525.

Bruni, M. (1998) *Fine Motor Skills in Children with Down Syndrome: A Guide For Parent and Professionals*. Bethesda MD: Woodbine Press.

Byrne, A., MacDonald, J., Buckley, S. (2002) Reading, language and memory skills: a comparative longitudinal study of children with Down syndrome and their mainstream peers. *Br J Educ Psychol*, **72**, 513–529.

Caselli, M. C., Vicari, S., Longobardi, E., Lami, L., Pizzoli, C., Stella, G. (1998) Gestures and words in early development of children with Down syndrome. *Journal of Speech, Language and Hearing Research*, **41**, 1125–1135.

Chapman, R. S. (1995) Language development in children and adolescents with Down syndrome. In P. Fletcher, B. MacWhinney (eds) *Handbook of Child Language*. Oxford: Blackwell, pp. 641–663.

Chapman, R. S., Seung, H. K., Schwartz, S. E., Kay-Raining Bird, E. (1998) Language skill of children and adolescents with Down syndrome: II. Production deficits. *Journal of Speech, Language, and Hearing Research*, **41**, 861–873.

Clibbens, J. (2001) Signing and lexical development in children with Down syndrome. *Down Syndrome: Research and Practice*, **7**, 101–105.

Clibbens, J., Powell, G. G., Atkinson, E. (2002) Strategies for achieving joint attention when signing to children with Down's syndrome. *International Journal of Language and Communication Disorders*, **37**, 309–323.

Cohen, W. I. (1999) Down syndrome: care of the child and family. In M. D. Levine, W. B. Carey, A. C. Crocker (eds), *Developmental-behavioral Pediatrics*, 3rd edn. Philadelphia: W. B. Saunders, pp. 240–248.

Cunningham, C. (1997) *Understanding Down Syndrome: An Introduction for Parents*. Cambridge MA: Brookline.

Foreman, P., Crews, G. (1998) Using augmentative communication with infants and young children with Down syndrome. *Down Syndrome: Research and Practice*, **5**, 16–25.

Gibson, D., Harris, A. (1988) Aggregated early intervention effects for Down's syndrome persons: patterning and longevity of benefits. *J Ment Defic Res*, **32**, 1–17.

Girolametto, L., Weitzman, E., Clements-Baartman, J. (1998) Vocabulary intervention for children with Down syndrome: parent training using focused stimulation. *Infant-Toddler Intervention*, **8**, 109–125.

Glenn, S., Dayus, B., Cunningham, C., Horgan, M. (2001) Mastery motivation in children with Down syndrome. *Down Syndrome: Research and Practice*, **7**, 52–59.

Guralnick, M. J. (ed.) (1997) *The Effectiveness of Early Intervention*. Baltimore:. Brookes.

Guralnick, M. J. (ed.) (2001) *Early Childhood Inclusion: Focus on Change*. Baltimore: Brookes.

Guralnick, M. J. (ed.) (2005) *Developmental Systems Approach to Early Intervention*. Baltimore: Brookes.

Hepburn, S. L. (2003) Clinical implications of temperamental characteristics of young children with developmental disabilities. *Infants and Young Children*, **16**, 59–76.

Hodapp, R. M., DesJardin, J. L., Ricci, L. A. (2003) Genetic syndromes of mental retardation: should they matter for the early interventionist? *Infants and Young Children*, **16**, 152–160.

Kim, J., Mahoney, G. (2004) The effects of mother's style of interaction on children's engagement: implications for using responsive interventions with parents. *Topics in Early Childhood Special Education*, **24**, 31–38.

Kumin, L., Von Hagel, K. C., Bahr, D. C. (2001) An effective oral motor intervention protocol for infants and toddlers with low muscle tone. *Infant-Toddler Intervention*, **11**, 181–200.

Landry, S. H., Miller-Loncar, C. L., Swank, P. R. (1998) Goal-directed behavior in children with Down syndrome: the role of joint play situations. *Early Education and Development*, **9**, 375–392.

Linn, M. I., Goodman, J. F., Lender, W. L. (2000) Played out? Passive behavior by children with Down syndrome during unstructured play. *Journal of Early Intervention*, **23**, 264–278.

Mahoney, G., Perales, F. (2005) Relationship-focused intervention with children with pervasive developmental disorders and other disabilities: a comparative study. *J Dev Behav Pediatr*, **26**, 77–85.

Mahoney, G., Perales, F. (2003) Using relationship-focused intervention to enhance the social-emotional functioning of young children with autism spectrum disorders. *Top Early Child Spec Educ*, **23**, 77–89.

McCathren, R. B., Yoder, P. J., Warren, S. F. (1995) The role of directives in early language intervention. *Journal of Early Intervention*, **19**, 91–101.

Moore, D. G., Oates, J. M., Hobson, R. P., Goodwin, J. (2002) Cognitive and social factors in the development of infants with Down syndrome. *Down Syndrome: Research and Practice*, **8**, 43–52.

National Education Goals Panel (NEGP) (1997) *Reconsidering Children's Early Development and Learning: Toward Common Views and Vocabulary*. Available at http://www.negp.gov/Reports/child-ea.htm.

Niccols, A., Atkinson, L., Pepler, D. (2003) Mastery motivation in young children with Down's syndrome: Relations with cognitive and adaptive competence. *J Intellect Disabil Res*, **47**, 121–133.

Pueschel, S. M., Pueschel, J. K. (eds) (1992) *Biomedical Concerns in Persons with Down Syndrome*. Baltimore MD: Brookes.

Ramruttun, B., Jenkins, C. (1998) Prelinguistic communication and Down syndrome. *Down Syndrome: Research and Practice*, **5**, 53–62.

Ratekin, C. (1996) Temperament in children with Down syndrome. *Dev Disabil Bull*, **24**, 18–32.

Roizen, N. J. (2003) The early interventionist and the medical problems of the child with Down syndrome. *Infants and Young Children*, **16**, 88–95.

Roper, N., Dunst, C. J. (2003) Communication interventions in natural environments: Guidelines for practice. *Infants and Young Children*, **16**, 215–226.

Sigman, M., Ruskin, E., Arbeile, S., Corona, R., Dissanayake, C., Espinosa, M. et al. (1999) Continuity and change in the social competence of children with autism, Down syndrome, and developmental delays. *Monogr Soc Res Child Dev*, **64**, 1–114.

Spiker, D., Boyce, G., Boyce, L. (2002) Parent-child interactions when infants and young children have disabilities. In L. Glidden (ed.) *International Review of Research in Mental Retardation*, Vol. 25. San Diego CA: Academic Press, pp. 35–70.

Spiker, D., Hebbeler, K. (1999) Early intervention services. In M. D. Levine et al. (eds) *Developmental-Behavioral Pediatrics*, 3rd edn. Philadelphia: Saunders, pp. 793–802.

Spiker, D., Hebbeler, K., Mallik, S. (2005) Developing and implementing early intervention programs: children with established disabilities. In M. J. Guralnick (ed.) *Developmental Systems Approach to Early Intervention*. Baltimore: Brookes.

Spiker, D., Hopmann, M. R. (1997) The effectiveness of early intervention for children with Down syndrome. In M. J. Guralnick (ed.) *The Effectiveness of Early Intervention*. Baltimore: Brookes, pp. 271–305.

Stores, R. (1993) A preliminary study of sleep disorders and daytime behaviour problems in children with Down syndrome. *Down Syndrome: Research and Practice*, **1**, 29–33.

VanDyke, D. C. (1995) *Medical and Surgical Care for Children with Down Syndrome: A Guide for Parents*. Bethesda MD: Woodbine.

Van Hooste, A., Maes, B. (2003) Family factors in the early development of children with Down syndrome. *Journal of Early Intervention*, **25**, 296–309.

Warren, S. F. (2000) The future of early communication and language intervention. *Topics in Early Childhood Special Education*, **20**, 33–37.

Winders, P. C. (1997) *Gross Motor Skills in Children with Down Syndrome: A Guide for Parents and Professionals*. Bethesda MD: Woodbine Press.

Wishart, J. (1993) The development of learning difficulties in children with Down's syndrome. *Journal of Intellectual Disability Research*, **37**, 389–403.

Wishart, J. (1996) Learning in young children with Down syndrome: Developmental trends. In J. A. Rondal, J. Perera (eds) *Down Syndrome: Psychological, Psychobiological, and Socio-educational Perspectives*. London: Whurr, pp. 81–96.

Wishart, J. (2001) Motivation and learning styles in young children with Down syndrome. *Down Syndrome: Research and Practice*, **7**, 47–51.

Yoder, P. J., Warren, S. F. (2004) Early predictors of language in children with and without Down syndrome. *Am J Ment Retard*, **109**, 285–300.

12 Family Setting in Down Syndrome

SALVATORE SORESI, LAURA NOTA, LEA FERRARI
University of Padua, Italy

SUMMARY

The birth of a child with Down syndrome (DS) requires the parents to revise their roles and to reconsider their tasks and activities. Throughout the life of the child, families have to cope with new situations that bring new challenges and fresh responsibilities. They need various forms of help and support.

Moreover, parents of DS children find themselves in a situation that is different in some respects from that of parents of children with other disabilities such as autism, sensory disabilities and emotional disorders. Effective strategies for managing family life can facilitate parental adjustment and increase the likelihood that parents will be able to foster greater development of adaptive competences in their own children. Service suppliers should take all these considerations into account when devising specific interventions in order to increase the probability that support and treatment will be effective.

INTRODUCTION

The birth of a child requires the adults in the family to revise their roles and to reconsider their tasks and activities, including reallocation of financial resources, to cope with the needs of the newcomer. When the child is born with DS the need for changes and adjustments becomes so pressing and stressful that one can think of this event as a turning point – a time when life significantly changes course (Seltzer et al. 2001; Soresi & Nota 2004). In time, families of individuals with DS have to cope with changes that, as well as creating new situations and bringing new challenges, require adjustments, fresh responsibilities and diverse forms of help and support.

Recent literature has privileged correlational analyses and transverse comparisons in analysing the situations these families have to deal with. In contrast, we have proposed a longitudinal and developmental perspective.

Down Syndrome: Neurobehavioural Specificity. Edited by JA Rondal and J Perera.
© 2006 John Wiley & Sons Ltd.

CHALLENGES AND TASKS THAT PARENTS OF A CHILD WITH DOWN SYNDROME HAVE TO FACE ACROSS THE LIFESPAN

At critical moments in their lives, parents of children with DS are exposed to complex situations that often require fresh energy and resources. This occurs, for instance, when they are told the diagnosis, during the early months and years of their child's life, during their child's school experiences from infancy to childhood, and the times when they have to deal with their adolescent child's requests and his or her transition to adulthood. Let us take a closer look at these 'critical times' and also reflect on the type of support that should be guaranteed by the local public health services.

PARENTS' CHALLENGES AND TASKS AT DIAGNOSIS

The point at which parents are told that their baby has been diagnosed with DS is their first real encounter with a situation that, until then, they have probably considered themselves highly unlikely to experience. The discomfort it can raise means that this is a problematic time that can significantly affect parents' early management of the child and also their future attitudes. The following reports (Van Riper et al. 1992), although highlighting some extreme experiences, can nevertheless be considered as representative of many parents' feelings at such times:

> the pediatrician entered the room and sat down with us, held our hands, and explained the best that he could what having such a child meant. He reassured us that this was a time for celebration, that she would make us happier than we could ever imagine and that the only thing that made her different was that one (lousy) chromosome. She would be able to do anything she wants (read, write, talk, walk, etc.), it might just take her a little longer than most. But give her time, you'll see . . . After his talk with us, I didn't cry anymore. I no longer felt sorry for myself. (Van Riper et al. 1992, p. 29)

> the only choices the doctor gave me were (1) I would take him home and love him. (2) put him in an institution. (3) order them to cut off his food supply . . . What no one told me and I desperately needed to hear, was that these children generate more love than is imaginable. I was scared to death of my baby . . . For the first few months, I felt suicidal. (Van Riper et al. 1992, p. 30)

The way health and social service providers tell parents the diagnosis and handle the first contacts with them is not always appropriate to the situation. For instance, Case (2001) reports that by far the great majority of parents of children born with impairment or disability would have preferred to have been told in a more professional way, with attention paid to the emotional state they were experiencing. They would have liked to have been treated in a more measured and personalised fashion. The majority of the parents stated that information necessary to understand the situation was seldom supplied directly; rather, it had to be expressly asked for. Moreover, the information was often incomplete, not up to date and lacking in terms of information about the consequences and likelihood of intervention in the short, medium and long term. Answers were often given in a 'technical' language that was not always easy to understand. Fox et al. (2002) report that the parents lamented the scarce information obtained from the services, as well as unclear, ambiguous and superficial indications (for example: 'your son will speak when he's ready'). Many of them stated that they had to look for other consultants themselves and search for further information by navigating the Internet, buying books and journals and trying to find other support, thus using a great deal of money, energy and resources.

PARENTS' CHALLENGES AND TASKS IN THEIR CHILD'S EARLY MONTHS AND YEARS

At a very early stage, parents of children with DS feel the need to have more time to care for their child, to take him or her for medical tests and special treatment – certainly more than parents of children without disability (Barnett & Boyce 1995; Padeliadu 1998). Because of the chronic health problems experienced by their children, the quality of the relationship between parents and professionals continues to be important (Leff & Walizer 1992).

However, given the great responsibility they have for their children's health, parents can obviously make errors and so attract criticism from health and social service providers, who tend to consider possible mistakes as the result of a lack of responsibility or, even worse, a lack of resolve and willingness (McDaniel et al. 1992). This kind of interaction typically entails discomfort, a sense of inadequacy, confusion, a lack of confidence in one's own educational abilities and sometimes even a sense of guilt, excessive self-devaluation, resentment and dissatisfaction (Thorne 1993). Very soon, some parents start to believe that they will never be able to obtain the help they need outside the family and they begin to have little confidence in the services, going so far as to avoid any relationship with health and social service providers. A belief that they can cope with their problems by themselves can encourage an increase in their expertise in managing their child's health but it can also curb their readiness to seek help when this is necessary. Van Riper (1999) specifically addressed the quality of the relationship between about 150 parents of DS children and health and social service providers. Considering the discrepancy between the 'ideal' relationship and the relationship that was actually experienced and the level of wellbeing and family functioning, the author showed that the lower such discrepancy was, the higher was the perceived level of satisfaction with the relationship and the greater was the propensity to ask health and social service providers for help. It was also associated with higher levels of parental wellbeing and better family functioning. What seemed to affect perception of low discrepancy more was health and social service providers' ability to pay attention to the family as a whole through actions that aimed to:

- adequately support difficulties and problems experienced by parents and family members each time new habilitation activities or new therapies were begun
- support the role that family members could have in the treatments of the child with disability
- support and adequately reinforce the efforts made and the decision processes activated by the family members themselves

PARENTS' CHALLENGES AND TASKS THROUGHOUT THEIR CHILDREN'S INFANCY AND CHILDHOOD

Evidence can easily be found in the literature that DS children's cognitive and social abilities can eventually be improved, even if at a slower pace than those of children without disability (Gibson 1978; Morgan 1979; Connolly et al. 1980; Sharav et al. 1985; Nadel 1988; Carr 1995; Hauser-Cram et al. 1999). Down syndrome children seem to have particular difficulties in communication and especially in expressive language (Smith & von Tetzchner 1986; Stoel-Gammon 1990; Chapman et al. 1991; Dykens et al. 1994; Rondal 2004); however, they have fewer difficulties in social development and in abilities associated with everyday tasks (Cornwell & Birch 1969; Tingey et al. 1991). Strengths and weaknesses may be different in each individual as he or she develops, even if typically there is a worsening of their existing deficits and an improvement in their strengths (Hodapp et al. 2003).

These are important findings that should be made known to parents and educators with the aim of encouraging suitable interventions. Fox et al. (2002) report that parents declared that, over a period of time, they had not received the support necessary to cope with their children's educational failures and the difficulties encountered in the everyday management of their children's general and behavioural problems. Abbeduto et al. (2001) maintain that children's learning is associated with the characteristics of their environment and that parents, in order to deal with educational tasks in such a way as to assist their children's cognitive and social development, should be able to have access to specific knowledge and to master educational skills that someone (the local services, we think) should have passed on to them. In children without disability, abilities functional to everyday life – such as washing, dressing and feeding themselves autonomously, talking, responding to school, family and social requests – develop without specific parental intervention. In children with disability, a great deal of instruction is needed: many exercises need to be carried out repeatedly and systematic attention must be given to the child in order to maintain and generalise results that are achieved with great effort (Lovaas 1983; Anderson et al. 1996). Parents, then, should be given guidance about how to spot their children's abilities and difficulties (they should be taught sophisticated observational strategies), how to plan specific interventions aiming at developing new skills, to use effective teaching techniques (such as instructions, suggestions, chaining, and modelling) to maintain the progress that has been made over a period of time (through reinforcement and negotiation) and to ensure that acquired abilities are generalised by controlling situations, stimuli and events and by adequately preparing the child's environment (Foxx 1982; Horner et al. 1988).

These educational interventions should diminish the 'natural tendency', typical of all family members, to stimulate only these children's strengths and would also encourage their ability to involve the children in tasks that would tax their less developed abilities (Hodapp et al. 2003). Specific knowledge on this tendency may also favour a more efficacious interaction with the educators and be useful to devise educational interventions that take into consideration all strengths and weaknesses and not only the most evident and easily identifiable ones (Fidler et al. 2003).

PARENTS' CHALLENGES AND TASKS DURING THEIR CHILDREN'S ADOLESCENCE AND EARLY ADULTHOOD

Like normally developing individuals, adolescents with DS wish to have friends of the same age, belong to their peer group, have opportunities for community life, have a job and be somewhat independent from their family (Calignano 2003a). However, social services cannot efficiently fulfil some of these wishes and, above all, cannot do it for all of these individuals (Jobling et al. 2000). At the end of compulsory schooling few adolescents with disability are included in a work setting; most of them end up spending a lot of time at home, or spend part of their day in day centres, socialising only with other disabled individuals (Soresi 2003). A mother writes:

As time goes by, many stimuli and interventions, especially the rehabilitative ones, dwindle into nothingness; once compulsory school is over most of these youths begin living under some sort of 'house isolation' to which they are not used. Suddenly they have no more engagements; they are in a sort of early retirement. It is as if they were told that all they have seen and experienced so far has only been to let them see how 'others' live. And these youths find themselves alone, without friends, without the chance of continuing their social inclusion, with parents who feel tired out, alone and without hope and enthusiasm. (Calignano 2003b, p. 127)

All this means a strain on their social network, spending most of their leisure time with their family and also receiving reduced support from care and rehabilitation professionals (Krauss & Erickson 1988). For the most part, these adolescents' social network is often made up of family members who find themselves playing various roles within it (for instance, a brother can carry out home management activities with the person with disability but he may also be the only person he or she confides in, or the one who takes care of transport needs, and so forth) and in which the mother holds a central position. These networks often involve individuals who belong to the mother's network; indeed 40% of them are her friends and so of the same age and gender as the mother (Krauss et al. 1992).

Some studies have clearly shown that, compared to individuals without disability, many young adults with DS do not have friends the same age as themselves (Buckley & Sacks 1987; Jobling 1989; Carr 1995) and that, in these cases, a favourite pastime is watching television. Many therefore begin to imagine 'friendships' with TV characters and think that interpersonal relationships are similar to those they see in soap operas – complex and dramatic, full of difficulties and hard to maintain in time (Jobling et al. 2000). Often, because of the lack of contacts outside the family, these young people experience a growing sense of depression and isolation that can make relationships within the family more difficult (Carr 1995).

On the other hand, as time goes by, mothers report feelings of fear, anxiety and uncertainty about their future and especially about the child's future. Many mothers feel that caregiving is their own personal responsibility and even when they realise that their difficulties are continually increasing they are reluctant to delegate some forms of support to other family members. This problem increases with time, with the loss of some members of the support network (Grant 1993).

PARENTS' CHALLENGES AND TASKS IN THEIR CHILDREN'S ADULTHOOD

Advances in medicine and in the health and social interventions typically carried out in Western societies have improved the health of individuals with DS and remarkably increased their life expectancy (Jenkins & MacDonald 2004). Until a few decades ago these individuals were thought to only exceptionally reach late adolescence or, at best, early adulthood; current estimates place their life expectancy at over 65 years for more than 15% of them and 55 years for more than 50% (Rondal 2004).

The increased longevity and the ageing processes of these individuals result in further pathologies and health problems that need to be addressed. In going from adolescence to adulthood, individuals with DS tend to become obese, experience problems associated to celiac disease and/or hypothyroidism (Annerén et al. 2004), have more severe eyesight problems because of cataracts (Prasher 1994) and suffer further hearing loss (Evenhuis et al. 1992). These individuals also show a marked predisposition to degenerative disorders like Alzheimer's disease (Wisniewski et al. 2004).

Family members therefore find themselves interacting with an adult individual hardly able to lead a completely independent life, to be economically self-sufficient and to autonomously organise his or her life. These individuals live mostly with their parents and continue to spend 8 hours a day either in occupational day centres or sheltered workshops. Feelings of loneliness and depression may persist or even worsen and mental health problems associated with early ageing can also emerge (Cooper 1997; Nota & Soresi 2002).

In addition to their child's ageing and worsening health, parents obviously find themselves having to deal with their own ageing, their own declining physical and motor abilities and a higher incidence of chronic illnesses that can make caring for the child more difficult (Seltzer & Krauss 1994). At this stage, parents should start to 'look around' and strive to find some solutions to the problem of providing care for the child after their own demise. However, only between 33% and 50% of elderly parents plan for the future; many hope that they will be able to continue to care for the child and this may imply not being ready to deal with the crisis situations that will inevitably occur (Bigby 2000).

Some parents tend to involve their other children who, in any case, may experience strong worries about their own and their sibling's future (Harland & Cuskelly 2000). It must also be considered that, in time, the instrumental support supplied by the siblings actually diminishes. They grow up and move away from the family home to lead an independent life of their own, leaving the parents with even greater responsibility as caregivers (Krauss et al. 1992; Greenberg et al. 1999; Harland & Cuskelly 2000; Perera 2004).

It follows that the services need to revise and update their counselling and support programmes in accordance with the changes under way. This requires a willingness to listen and a propensity to revise routine ways of responding to parents and families in the light of new and emerging difficulties (Perera 1995).

SPECIFICITY OF PARENTS OF CHILDREN WITH DS

Parents of children with DS, from the very beginning, have to reconsider their family organisation and give stronger support in response to specific requests for help made by a child with intellectual disability. They very soon become aware that they must cope with a condition that is different from their expectations. Parents of children with problems due to autism or to sensory disabilities only begin to realise that 'something is wrong' and that they have to cope with the problems associated with those disabilities later on, usually during the first years of their child's development. Emotional and psychological difficulties, like schizophrenia or other intellectual disabilities, usually appear during late infancy or adolescence, which means that parents begin to experience a lower level of wellbeing and greater psychological discomfort only after years of educational relationships with their children (Seltzer et al. 2001; Seltzer et al. 2004).

Parents of children with DS and with autism usually find themselves having to cope with disability problems in their young adulthood, while those with children with schizophrenia and other psychological disorders cope with them in their middle age. Moreover, in the first stages of autism and of schizophrenia, behavioural problems, which are less evident and less intense in their peers with DS, appear very frequently. The latter's maladaptive behaviours are usually fairly constant across the lifespan and as time goes by do not typically present sudden changes as regards frequency, intensity and noxiousness (Zigman et al. 1994). Maladaptive behaviours of individuals with autism are often far less stable: initially they are very severe and tend to either decrease or increase with age (Seltzer et al. 2000). In this connection, Holmes & Carr (1991) showed that at least three-quarters of the parents they interviewed who had children with DS stated that their child was easier to manage as an adult, while at least half the parents of children with autism reported greater problems in managing an adult child. Schizophrenia seems to have a more cyclic and less predictable trend: some individuals show difficulties in middle and late adulthood and others present either a constant course or a steady worsening (Harding 1988).

Pelchat et al. (1999), for instance, have found that parents of children with palatoschisis and parents of children with DS, despite having to deal with a situation different from expectations from the very beginning and experiencing very similar levels of stress and emotional discomfort, do present differences in parental adjustment over time. If the former see their difficulties reduce in time due to appropriate surgery, the latter acquire an increasing awareness of their children's difficulties and feel increasing need for further support.

Other studies illustrate that parents of children with DS seem to show a lesser tendency to develop a different image of themselves, their children, and their families, as compared with parents of children with autism or sensory disabilities. The authors go so far as to say that parents that cope with greater and more manifest disabilities may find forming more positive child, parent, and family images a more complex task (Wilgosh et al. 2004; Nota et al. 2005).

Service providers should take this into account if they intend to devise specific interventions to increase the probability that support and treatment will be effective (Nota 2004; Soresi 2004). Although research in this field is still necessary, it is clear that the 'parental world' appears particularly complex and varied for these parents. If the difficulties of parents and families that live in daily contact with disability are to be eased it will be increasingly necessary to use up-to-date specific knowledge and to abandon generic, simplistic, superficial, standardised visions and assumptions. In other words, as different disabilities are addressed through different health, pharmacological, habilitation and rehabilitation interventions and different forms of counselling, 'parental differences' will also have to be dealt with via heterogeneous modalities of support and training.

This is evident when other specific differences are considered that would seem to characterise the families of individuals with disability and, in particular, with DS: communication styles and family climates.

Mink et al. (1983), for instance, studied 115 families of children with disability and showed that the children who lived in cohesive and harmonious families had better socio-emotional functioning. Mink & Nihira (1986) underscored that family cohesion affected the psychological adjustment of adolescents with learning difficulties. A series of studies on individuals with DS revealed that high levels of cohesion were predictors of higher motivation to do school tasks (Hauser-Cram 1993) and of more positive school interactions with peers (Hauser-Cram et al. 1997). Moreover, positive interactions between mother and child (both with typical development and with disability) are associated with the child acquiring better cognitive and communication abilities (Barnard 1997).

These data are also important given that children with intellectual disability, including DS, can be less responsive social partners for their parents, especially in early infancy, as they tend to have less social initiative: they initiate fewer interactions and produce fewer clearly identifiable social actions than children with typical development (Spiker & Hopmann 1997).

Hauser-Cram et al. (1999) studied 54 children with DS (mean age about 3 years) and their family members. During their 5-year longitudinal research, they examined the children's adaptive behaviour and their psychomotor development, the mother-child interaction modalities in teaching tasks and family cohesion. The authors found that the children under observation, who initially had the same level of adaptive functioning and psychomotor development, with time showed rhythms of adaptive development related to quality of family relationships. In particular, it appeared that family relationships predicted the development of communication, social and everyday abilities. Family cohesiveness and the ability of mothers of children with DS to have emotionally supportive interactions, to react responsively to their children and to propose situations for teaching cognitive skills favour the adaptive development of their children with DS.

Pelchat et al. (2003) maintained that fathers seem to show lower levels of sensitivity than mothers and that the difference is more marked the more severe the disability is. Parental sensitivity was defined as the parent's ability to perceive and accurately interpret the child's signals and to respond to them adequately and promptly. Furthermore, Pelchat et al. said that fathers react in a more negative way to cognitive disabilities, which agrees with those studies illustrating the tendency of fathers to consider problems connected with their children's cognitive abilities especially negatively. For instance, Renaud et al. (1993) showed that, among Canadian doctors interested in the new reproductive techniques, men were more in favour than women of selective abortion when DS was diagnosed whereas this difference did not emerge when a sensory or motor disability was diagnosed. Pelchat et al. maintain that fathers' lower sensitivity could also be related to their lower ability to decipher the child's signals, due perhaps to their spending less time than mothers interacting with the child.

These abilities can be considered as 'emotional' and 'relational' coping strategies. The former involve the ability to express one's feelings and emotions openly, to 'stop' the tendency to excite negative feelings in oneself and in others, to resort to negotiation in moments of conflict, to take into consideration the needs of the other family members, of one's partner and children without disability. 'Relational' strategies concern the ability to pay close attention to family cohesion, to the development of adaptive abilities in family members and to cooperation and tolerance (Burr & Klein 1994; Soresi & Nota 2004). These strategies should be associated with cognitive strategies that refer to the 'reformulation' of what has happened, to finding some positive aspects despite everything, to revisiting one's experience in the light of more detailed information and scientific knowledge (Burr & Klein 1994). Reformulation should also include one's own personal objectives. When a baby is on the way, parents actually set objectives for themselves – about things that can be done all together, about the help that a child can give his/her parents once they have become old, and so forth – and for the child, too: what he or she will do when he or she grows up and so on. Personal objectives can help significantly to organise one's experiences and stimulate parents to realise what is necessary to pursue them, thus favouring the achievement of higher levels of satisfaction (Emmons 1999). However, when life circumstances change greatly and situations arise in which the expected objectives can no longer be pursued, continuing to focus attention on them can cause anguish and depression. In this regard, King & Patterson (2000) asked 87 parents of children with DS first to describe how they had imagined their life before becoming the parents of a child with DS – what they had dreamed and hoped for – then the authors asked them what they had thought about their future life after the birth of the child and what they thought could now be their 'best possible life'. The parents filled out some questionnaires on emotional wellbeing, experienced moods and perceived stress. The parents who were successful in reviewing their objectives had 'grown' more following their experience of having a baby with DS and had become better able to deal with stressful situations. This confirms that individuals are more inclined to use active coping strategies if they believe that their hopes for the future can be realised (Taylor & Armor 1996). Sense of personal growth is also related to keeping in mind the objectives that had been set in the past, without it nega-tively affecting level of wellbeing; personal growth can actually occur only when losses are also analysed and recognised. It would seem that happiness and personal growth follow two somewhat different routes: the former due to revisiting one's own objectives, the latter due to reflections on what has been lost and what has been gained. Parents of children with DS can satisfy their original objectives, or at least some of them, if they have other children and they can also experience personal advantages not envisaged before. This can make the sense of loss less negative when compared with other situations, for example a divorce (King et al. 2000).

WHAT CAN THE SERVICES DO AND WHAT SHOULD THEY BE MORE INSISTENTLY ASKED TO DO?

We have tried, within an essentially developmental perspective, to illustrate the challenges and difficult tasks that parents of children with disability – specifically with DS – have to face across the lifespan. We have also tried to indicate the type of support that they would need and highlighted the fact that services and interventions to help these families should be personalised, specific and in line with the different challenges confronting them.

It is clear that it is not enough to focus only on the child or adolescent with difficulty; it is also necessary to promote family cohesion and positive rela-tionships between parents and between them and their children. Assessment activities should not privilege only disabilities, impairments, 'activity restric-tions' and cognitive deficits; they should also carefully consider parental resources, their knowledge and the abilities of parents and of family members. Problems of family isolation, reduced social networks, scarce family cohesion and failure to use social skills that are useful for encouraging positive and responsive relationships should alarm service suppliers and alert them to the need to intervene. We are convinced that healthcare services experienced in assessment and personalised interventions can probably make the difference with families at risk.

The final part of this chapter will be devoted to this issue in the hope that the services will, on the one hand, show greater attention to specific needs and demands and, on the other, be increasingly open to genuine forms of participation, involvement and collaboration.

First of all, it is important to remember that over the last few years there have been a number of research studies that seem to indicate that these parents, after a short period of bewilderment, actually 'roll up their sleeves', make strong efforts and can frequently cope with their problems surprisingly well. Some studies seem to go so far as to emphasise that the relationship between an adult with disability and his/her parents encourages parents' perception of wellbeing (Rossi & Rossi 1990; Townsend & Franks 1995;

Blieszner & Bedford 1996; Li 2000). In the literature there is no major evidence that having a child with DS automatically produces negative effects on the family system, whether at conjugal or parental level, or on the other family members (Perera 2004). The parents of children with DS seem to show the same levels of quality of life and self-efficacy beliefs as the parents of children with sensory disability and with typical development (Nota et al. 2005). Despite everything, the parents of children with developmental disabilities like DS or autism seem to share the idea that their commitment in caring for their children has made them develop strengths and acceptance of life events they would have never developed otherwise (Krauss & Seltzer 2000). Greenberg et al. (2004) indicated that parents of adults with DS show the same levels of optimism and health as other groups of parents of children with difficulties.

Moreover, in addition to the differences that can be seen between parents of children with diverse disabilities and which must obviously be carefully considered, the fact remains that they all share very demanding educational tasks. On that basis the services can also think about preventive interventions that could be more general and useful, independently of the type of disability dealt with.

The services should implement support programmes that recognise the great importance of the ways in which diagnosis, and possible prognosis are communicated by envisaging:

- an accurate description of the first difficulties parents will have to cope with and also of the progress the child might make
- using operational language that is as clear as possible and that is in line with parents' schooling and their knowledge about disability so that the information is easily understood by the individuals concerned
- unhurried interviews, carried out by professionals with a serious but relaxed attitude, during which parents can ask all the important questions they have and obtain useful answers and suggestions on how to manage the child's early life

Another aspect of the quality of the services supplied concerns the ability to initiate systematic parent involvement. Following communication of the diagnosis, further meetings between parents and specifically trained personnel should be arranged to assess some of the parents' characteristics (communication abilities, coping strategies, educational abilities) and to facilitate the counselling and training necessary to strengthen some of their educational competences (Case 2000, 2001).

As mentioned above, it may be important, when needed, to provide parents with specific educational skills that will be useful for the child's early development and to help them collaborate with the services to facilitate timely linguistic, motor and cognitive interventions (Soresi & Nota 2004).

During child development and throughout the lifespan of individuals with disability, the services should encourage the greatest possible autonomy and integration. As regards school-age children, it would be important for services not only to stimulate maintenance of parents' educational abilities but also to work actively to encourage integration and especially school inclusion (Nota & Soresi 2004). We think that the services are shirking their responsibility when they accept that some parents continue to prefer sending their children, for their 'happiness' and 'security', to institutionalised centres, which are sheltered and therefore overprotective. Parents should be encouraged to aim for complete inclusion, even if it entails added difficulties and some risks. They should be supported in this with actions that totally remove the risk of segregation and make schools increasingly integrating places.

As far as adolescents with DS are concerned, the end of compulsory schooling represents one of the most significant moments in their lives and in those of their families. Only a very few 'lucky' ones will begin professional activities in normal settings. It therefore becomes crucial to provide forms of support that aim to create opportunities for social, community and work inclusion, which support parents in their effort of encouraging their child's social life, and which teach parents to manage worrying behaviours (for example, in the sexual sphere) (Del Re & Bazzo 1997; Bazzo et al., in press) and that prevent the 'stagnating' of family relationships (Nota & Soresi 1997). The most significant is without a doubt guaranteeing work inclusion, as work encourages the development of professional identity and, consequently, the wider development of personal identity (Vondracek & Skorikov 1997; Soresi & Nota 2000; Soresi & Nota 2003).

In this regard, collaboration with parents is very important and particular attention has to be paid to their attitudes. Some may find it difficult to realise that their children are growing up; some tend to think that work is only a way to keep them 'busy', to have little confidence in their childrens' productive abilities, or perhaps they might discourage work inclusion because they are afraid to lose their pension rights. Such parents can think, along with other people in society, that their children with DS are 'eternal children' and so they ask their employer not to tire them too much, or ask whether they can 'have more holidays', without thinking that in doing so their children are likely to be thought unable to play a significant role at the workplace, debasing their social image as workers (Contardi 2003).

The services should take parents' wishes into consideration and envisage specific instructional and educational activities centred on the reconceptualisation of work in individuals with disabilities in order to help parents to promote greater self-determination in adult life and to encourage and maintain successful work inclusion.

For adults, it is important to focus on training and supporting parents in the transition from situations in which they have the main caring role to situations where the person with DS is either cared for in residential structures or by other family members. The planning of this event is rather complex: parents often show discomfort and difficulty in thinking about their children's future. The services themselves have little experience in this area and they have often not established proper relationships with the other family members over time (Bigby 2000). Sometimes, parents find it hard to approach the services because of unhappy previous experiences, negative attitudes toward themselves and interactions that only led to a sense of guilt and discomfort. They have lost faith in the likelihood of having helpful answers to their needs (Stehlik 1997).

The planning that we are advocating here is a way of guaranteeing greater security and stability to individuals with intellectual disability and anticipating the best answers to their needs. If it is carried out it can guarantee greater psychological wellbeing for parents, too (Kaufman et al. 1991). The planning should involve three particularly important fields: social security, financial resources and housing.

An efficient intervention for elderly parents should involve:

• monitoring of situations in which there are elderly family members who will have to be considered as possible users of health and social services
• initiatives involving parents in the planning of future projects, so as to avoid improvident and inadequately planned transition situations
• analysis of the possible future needs of the individual with disability
• preparing adults with intellectual disability for the different 'transitions' they will encounter
• providing support to parents so that they can continue with their role of caregivers as long as possible
• providing counselling and psychological support to parents to enable them to manage the conflict situations they experience during these transitions in the best possible way and to successfully renegotiate their roles (Wood 1993; Kelly & Kropf 1995; Smith et al. 1995; Janicki 1996)

Finally, special attention should be paid to family cohesion and to social skills that help to encourage positive and responsive relationships within the family. Pelchat et al. (1999), for instance, carried out interventions with parents of children with DS immediately after their birth, involving all the family, highlighting the strengths and the adaptive abilities of the family and of all its members. The aim was to encourage family autonomy and empowerment and to optimise existing resources and the adjustment of the different members. In particular, the aims were to:

• identify each parent's perceptions and opinions about having a baby with DS
• encourage revision of the less advantageous and adaptive ones and strengthen those that favour adjustment

- make the couple understand each other's feelings about the situation and become able to support each other to overcome their grief and to encourage adjustment processes
- help parents to have significant relationships with people outside the family and use the resources available and the help of social and healthcare operators more efficiently

The programme, which envisaged between six and eight meetings – two immediately after the birth of the child and the others at home during the following 6 months – proved capable of helping parents to adjust better in the first 18 months of the child's life. In addition, the parents who had participated in the activity had a lower level of parental stress and emotional suffering compared with those who had not participated; they reported perceiving a higher level of emotional support from their partners and felt more confident in the help they would receive from others.

Soresi & Nota (2004) have also devised a parent training intervention over 14 meetings aiming to strengthen coping strategies, problem-solving abilities and assertive abilities. Parents who have benefited from such interventions show increments in levels of knowledge of educational principles and levels of wellbeing and satisfaction (Soresi 1998; Soresi & Nota 2004).

The success of these parent training interventions depends on them being carried out as early as possible and involving the children's fathers. Improving parent's relationship skills and providing them with more accurate knowledge of their children's disability can also encourage a more effective use of health and social resources. It is necessary to maintain and generalise these skills and knowledge to help parents keep cohesion and harmony in the family over time and to help them to cope effectively with the demanding tasks involved in the education and care of a growing child.

Service providers should supply a service that takes into account parents' abilities, emotional and cognitive skills and values. This would allow parents to be active agents participating in the decisions that have to be made as regards their children, conscious collaborators and also 'lively' supporters of their own rights and those of their children.

REFERENCES

Abbeduto, I., Evans, J., Dolan, T. (2001) Theoretical perspectives on language and communication in mental retardation and developmental disabilities. *Ment Retard Dev Disabil Res Rev*, **7**, 45–55.

Anderson, S. R., Taras, M., O'Malley Cannon, B. (1996) Teaching new skills to young children with autism. In C. Maurice, G. Green, S. C. Luce (eds) *Behavioral Intervention for Young Children with Autism. A Manual for Parents and Professionals*. Austin TX: Pro Ed, pp. 181–194.

Annerén, G., Myrelid, Å., Gustafsson, J. (2004) Growth retardation in Down syndrome: thyroid disorders, coeliac disease and the effect of GH therapy. In J. A. Rondal, A. Rasore Quartino, S. Soresi (eds) *The Adult with Down Syndrome. A New Challenge for Society.* London: Whurr, pp. 61–66.

Barnard, K. E. (1997) Influencing parent-child interactions for children at risk. In M. J. Guralnick (ed.) *The Effectiveness of Early Intervention.* Baltimore: Brookes, pp. 249–268.

Barnett, W. S., Boyce, G. C. (1995) Effects of children with Down syndrome on parent's activities. *Am J Ment Retard,* **100,** 115–127.

Bazzo, G., Nota, L., Soresi, S., Ferrari, L., Minnes, P. (in press) Attitudes of social service providers toward the sexuality of individuals with intellectual disability. *J Appl Res Intellect Disabil.*

Bigby, C. (2000) *Moving On without Parents.* Sydney: Maclennan & Petty.

Blieszner, R., Bedford, V. H. (1996) *Aging and the Family: Theory and Research.* Westport CT: Praeger.

Buckley, S., Sacks, B. (1987) *The Adolescent with Down's Syndrome: Life for the Teenager and For the Family.* Portsmouth UK: Portsmouth Polytechnic.

Burr, W. R., Klein, S. R. (1994) *Reexamining Family Stress. New Theory and Research.* London: Sage.

Calignano, M. T. (2003a) L'organizzazione scolastica per l'accoglienza e l'integrazione del disabile [School organisation: welcoming and including individuals with disabilities]. In M. Gelati, M. T. Calignano (eds) *Progetti di vita per le persone con sindrome di Down [Life Projects for Down Syndrome Persons].* Pisa: Edizioni Del Cerro, pp. 28–40.

Calignano, M. T. (2003b) Sindrome di Down e vita adulta [Down syndrome and adult life]. In M. Gelati, M. T. Calignano (eds) *Progetti di vita per le persone con sindrome di Down [Life Projects for Down Syndrome Persons].* Pisa: Edizioni del Cerro, pp. 125–133.

Carr, J. (1995) *Down's Syndrome: Children Growing Up.* Cambridge UK: Cambridge University Press.

Case, S. (2000) Refocusing on the parent: what are the social issues of concern for parents of disabled children? *Disability and Society,* **15,** 271–292.

Case, S. (2001) Learning to partner, disabling conflict: early indications of an improving relationship between parents and professionals with regard to service provision for children with disabilities. *Disability and Society,* **16,** 837–854.

Chapman, R., Schwartz, S., Kay-Raining Bird, E. (1991) Fast-mapping in stories: deficits in Down's syndrome. Communication at the Annual Meeting of the American Speech-Language-Hearing Association. Atlanta GA, November.

Connolly, B., Morgan, S., Russell, F., Richardson, B. (1980) Early intervention with Down's syndrome children: a follow-up report. *Phys Ther,* **60,** 1405–1408.

Contardi, A. (2003) Le persone con sindrome di Down al lavoro: esperienze e riflessioni nel cammino dell'Associazione Italiana Persone Down [Down syndrome individuals at work: experiences and thoughts of the Italian Association of Down Syndrome Individuals]. In M. Gelati, M. T. Calignano (eds), *Progetti di vita per le persone con sindrome di Down [Life Projects for Down Syndrome Persons].* Pisa: Edizioni Del Cerro, pp. 113–124.

Cooper, S. (1997) Deficient health and social services for elderly people with learning disabilities. *J Intellect Disabil Res,* **41,** 331–338.

Cornwell, A. C., Birch, H. G. (1969) Psychological and social development in home-reared children with Down's syndrome. *Am J Ment Defic*, **74**, 341–350.

Del Re, G., Bazzo, G. (1997) *Educazione sessuale e relazionale-affettiva. Scuola Media Superiore [Sexual and Social Education for High School Students]*. Trento: Erickson Editrice.

Dykens, E. M., Hodapp, R. M., Evans, D. W. (1994) Profiles and development of adaptive behavior in children with Down Syndrome. *Am J Ment Retard*, **98**, 580–587.

Emmons, R. A. (1999) *The Psychology of Ultimate Concerns: Motivation and Spirituality in Personality*. New York: Guilford.

Evenhuis, H. M., Van Zanten, G. A., Brocaar, M. P., Roerdinkholder, W. H. M. (1992) Hearing loss in middle-age in persons with Down's syndrome. *Am J Ment Retard*, **97**, 47–56.

Fidler, D. J., Lawson, J. E., Hodapp, R. M. (2003) What do parents want? An analysis of education-related comments made by parents of children with different genetic syndromes. *J Intellect Dev Disabil*, **28**, 196–204.

Fox, L., Vaughn, B. J., Llanes Wyatte, M., Dunlap, G. (2002) 'We can't expect other people to understand': family perspectives on problem behavior. *Exceptional Children*, **68**, 437–450.

Foxx, R. M. (1982) *Decreasing Behaviors of Persons with Severe Retardation and Autism*. Champaign IL: Research Press.

Gibson, D. (1978) *Down's Syndrome: The Psychology of Mongolism*. Cambridge UK: Cambridge University Press.

Grant, G. (1993) Support networks and transitions over two years among adults with mental handicap. *Mental Handicap Research*, **6**, 36–55.

Greenberg, J. S., Seltzer, M. M., Krauss, W. M., Chou, R. J., Hong, J. (2004) The effect of quality of the relationship between mothers and adult children with schizophrenia, autism or Down syndrome on maternal well-being: the mediating role of optimism. *Am J Orthopsychiatry*, **74**, 14–25.

Greenberg, J. S., Seltzer, M. M., Orsmond, G. I., Krauss, M. W. (1999) Siblings of adults with mental illness or mental retardation: influences on current involvement and the expectations of future caregiving responsiblity. *Psychiatr Serv*, **50**, 1214–1219.

Harding, C. M. (1988) Course types in schizophrenia: an analysis of European and American studies. *Schizophr Bull*, **14**, 633–643.

Harland, P., Cuskelly, M. (2000) The responsibilities of adults siblings of adults with dual sensory impairments. *Int J Disabil Dev Educ*, **47**, 293–307.

Hauser-Cram, P. (1993) Mastery motivation in three-year-old children with Down syndrome. In D. J. Messer (ed.) *Mastery Motivation: Children's Investigation, Persistence and Development*. London: Routledge, pp. 230–250.

Hauser-Cram, P., Warfield, M., Bronson, M. B., Krauss, M. W., Shonkoff, J. P., Upshur, C. C. (1997) Family influence on changes in school competence of young children with Down syndrome. Paper presented at the biennial meeting of the Society for Research in Child Development, Washington DC, April.

Hauser-Cram, P., Warfield, M., Shonkoff, J., Krauss, M. W., Upshur, C. C., Sayer, A. (1999) Family influence on adaptive development in young children with Down syndrome. *Child Dev*, **70**, 979–989.

Hodapp, R. M., DesJardin, J., Ricci, L. A. (2003) Genetic syndromes of mental retardation. Should they matter for the early interventionist? *Infant and Young Children*, **16**, 152–160.

Holmes, N., Carr, J. (1991) The pattern of care in families of adults with a mental handicap. A comparison between families of autistic adults and Down syndrome adults. *J Autism Dev Disord*, **2**, 159–176.

Horner, R. H., Dunlap, G., Koegel, R. L. (1988) *Generalization and Maintenance: Life-style Changes in Applied Settings*. Baltimore, Paul Brookes.

Janicki, M. (1996) *Help for Caring for Older People Caring for Adults with a Developmental Disability*. Albany NY: New York State Developmental Disabilities Planning Council.

Jenkins, C., MacDonald, J. (2004) Developing the language skills of adults with Down syndrome. In J. A. Rondal, A. Rasore Quartino, S. Soresi (eds) *The Adult with Down Syndrome. A New Challenge for Society*. London: Whurr.

Jobling, A. (1989) Leisure, recreation and residence. In P. Gunn, J. Bramley (eds) *Adolescent Girls with Intellectual Disabilities: School and Post-school Options*. St Lucia, Queensland: The University of Queensland, Fred and Eleanor Schonell Special Education Research Centre, pp. 89–100.

Jobling, A., Moni, K. B., Nolan, A. (2000) Understanding friendship: young adults with Down syndrome exploring relationships. *J Intellect Disabil*, **25**, 235–245.

Kaufman, A., Adams, J., Campbell, V. (1991) Permanency planning by older parents who care for adult children with mental retardation. *Ment Retard*, **29**, 293–300.

Kelly, T., Kropf, N. (1995) Stigmatised and perpetual parents: older parents caring for adult children with lifelong disabilities. *Journal of Gerontological Social Work*, **20**, 3–16.

King, L. A., Patterson, C. (2000) Reconstructing life goals after the birth of a child with Down syndrome: finding happiness and growing. *Int J Rehabil Health*, **5**, 17–30.

King, L. A., Ramsey, C. M., Smith, N. G., Bell, C. G. (2000) Lost and Found Possible Selves, Subjective Well-being and Ego Development. Unpublished manuscript. Dallas TX: Southern Methodist University.

Krauss, M., Erickson, M. (1988) Informal support networks among aging person with mental retardation. A pilot study. *Ment Retard*, **26**, 197–201.

Krauss, M. W., Seltzer, M. M. (2000) An unanticipated life: the impact of lifelong caregiving. In H. Bersani (ed.) *Responding to the Challenge: International Trends and Current Issues in Developmental Disabilities*. Brookline MA: Brookline Books, pp. 173–188.

Krauss, M. W., Seltzer, M. M., Goodman, S. J. (1992) Social support networks of adults with mental retardation who live at home. *Am J Ment Retard*, **96**, 432–441.

Leff, P., Walizer, E. (1992) *Building the Healing Partnership: Parents, Professional, and Children with Chronic Illnesses and Disabilities*. New York: Brookline.

Li, L. (2000) Intergenerational Relationships and Psychological Well-being of Mildlife Daughters. Unpublished doctoral dissertation, University of Wisconsin – Madison.

Lovaas, O. I. (1983) *Teaching Developmentally Disabled Children: The ME Book*. Austin TX: Pro-Ed.

McDaniel, S. H., Hepworth, J., Doherty, W. J. (1992) *Medical Family Therapy: A Biopsychosocial Approach to Families with Health Problems*. New York: Basic Books.

Mink, I. T., Nihira, K. (1986) Family life–styles and child behaviors: a study of direction of effects. *Dev Psychol*, **22**, 610–616.

Mink, I. T., Nihira, K., Meyers, C. E. (1983) Taxonomy of family life styles: 1. Homes with TMR children. *Am J Ment Defic*, **87**, 484–497.

Morgan, S. B. (1979) Development and distribution of intellectual and adaptive skills in Down syndrome children. *Ment Retard*, **17**, 247–249.

Nadel, L. (1988) *The Psychobiology of Down Syndrome*. Cambridge MA: MIT Press.

Nota, L. (2004) Family involvement in the treatment of individuals with intellectual disability. In J. A. Rondal, A. Rasore Quartino, S. Soresi (eds) *The Adult with Down Syndrome. A New Challenge for Society*. London: Whurr Publishers, pp. 205–211.

Nota, L., Soresi, S. (1997) *I comportamenti sociali: dall'analisi all'intervento. [Social Behaviors: from Analysis to Intervention]*. Pordenone: Erip Editrice.

Nota, L., Soresi, S. (2002) Psicopatalogia e ritardo mentale [Psychopathology and mental retardation]. In S. Soresi (ed.) *Disabilità, trattamento, integrazione*. Pordenone: Erip.

Nota, L., Soresi, S. (2004) Social and community inclusion. In J. Rondal, R. Hodapp, S. Soresi, E. Dykens, L. Nota (eds) *Intellectual Disabilities. Genetics, Behaviour, and Inclusion*. London: Whurr, pp. 157–192.

Nota, L., Soresi, S., Ferrari, L., Wilgosh, L., Scorgie, K. (2005) Life Management and quality of life of parents of children with diverse disabilities. *Dev Disabil Bull*, **31**, 155–181.

Padeliadu, S. (1998) Time demands and stress in Greek mothers of children with Down syndrome. *J Intellect Disabil Res*, **42**, 144–153.

Pelchat, D., Bisson, J., Bois, C., Saucier, J. F. (2003) The effects of early relational antecedents and other factors on the parental sensitivity of mothers and fathers. *Infant Child Dev*, **12**, 27–51.

Pelchat, A., Bisson, J., Richard, N., Perreault, M., Bouchard, J. M. (1999) Longitudinal effects of an early family intervention programme on the adaptation of parents of children with a disability. *Int J Nurs Stud*, **36**, 465–477.

Perera, J. (1995) *Síndrome de Down. Aspectos específicos*. Barcelona: Masson.

Perera, J. (2004) Siblings in the family of a person with Down syndrome. In J. A. Rondal, A. Rasore Quartino, S. Soresi (eds) *The Adult with Down Syndrome. A New Challenge for Society*. London: Whurr, pp. 194–204.

Prasher, V. (1994) Screening of ophthalmic pathology and its associated effects on adaptive behaviour in adults with Down's syndrome. *Eur J Psychiatr*, **8**, 197–204.

Renaud, M., Bouchard, L., Bisson, J., Labadie, J. F., Dallaire, L., Kishchuck, N. (1993) Canadian physicians and prenatal diagnosis: prudence and ambivalence. In *Current Practice of Prenatal Diagnosis in Canada*, Vol. 13. Ottawa: Government of Canada, pp. 235–507.

Rondal, J. A. (2004) Language in adults with Down syndrome. In J. A. Rondal, A. Rasore Quartino, S. Soresi (eds) *The Adult with Down Syndrome. A New Challenge for Society*. London: Whurr Publisher, pp. 148–159.

Rossi, A. S., Rossi, P. H. (1990) *Of Human Bonding: Parent-child Relations Across the Life Course*. New York: Aldine de Gruyter.

Seltzer, M. M., Abbeduto L., Krauss, M. W., Greenberg, J., Swe, A. (2004) Comparison groups in autism family research: Down syndrome, fragile X syndrome and schizophrenia. *J Autism Dev Disord*, **34**, 41–48.

Seltzer, M. M., Greenberg, J. S., Floyd, F. J., Pettee, Y., Hong, J. (2001) Life course impact of parenting a child with disabilities. *Am J Ment Retard*, **106**, 265–286.

Seltzer, M. M., Krauss, M. W. (1994) Aging parents with co-resident adult children: the impact of lifelong caregiving. In M. Seltzer, M. Krauss, M. Janicki (eds) *Life Course Perspectives on Adulthood and Old Age*. Washington DC: American Association on Mental Retardation, pp. 3–18.

Seltzer, M. M., Krauss, M. W., Orsmond, G. I., Vestal, C. (2000) Families of adolescents and adults with autism: Uncharted territory. In L. M. Glidden (ed.) *International Review of Research on Mental Retardation*, Vol. 23, San Diego CA: Academic Press, pp. 267–294.

Sharav, T., Collins, R., Shlomo, L. (1985) Effect of maternal education on prognosis of development in children with Down syndrome. *Pediatrics*, **76**, 387–391.

Smith, L., Von Tetzchner, S. (1986) Communicative, sensorimotor and language skills of young children with Down syndrome. *Am J Ment Defic*, **91**, 57–66.

Smith, T. E. C., Polloway, E. A., Patton, J. R., Dowdy, C. A. (1995) *Teaching Students with Exceptional Needs in Inclusive Settings*. Boston: Allyn & Bacon.

Soresi, S. (1998) *Psicologia dell'handicap e della riabilitazione [Psychology of Handicap and Rehabilitation]*. Bologna: Il Mulino.

Soresi, S. (2003) *Disabilità, trattamento, integrazione [Disability, Treatment, Inclusion]*. Pordenone: Erip.

Soresi, S. (2004) Evaluating treatment outcomes. In J. A. Rondal, A. Rasore Quartino, S. Soresi (eds) *The Adult with Down Syndrome. A New Challenge for Society*. London: Whurr, pp. 235–250.

Soresi, S., Nota, L. (2000) A social skill training for persons with Down's Syndrome. *Eur Psychol*, **1**, 34–43.

Soresi, S., Nota, L. (2003) *Parent training per genitori di figli disabili [Parent Training for Parents of Children with Disability]*. Roma: Carocci Editore.

Soresi, S., Nota, L. (2004) School inclusion. In J. Rondal, R. Hodapp, S. Soresi, E. Dykens, L. Nota (eds) *Intellectual Disabilities. Genetics, Behaviour, and Inclusion*. London: Whurr Publishers Limited, pp. 114–156.

Spiker, D., Hopmann, M. R. (1997) The effectiveness of early intervention for children with Down syndrome. In M. J. Guralnick (ed.) *The Effectiveness of Early Intervention*. Baltimore: Brookes, pp. 271–305.

Stehlik, D. (1997) Learning to be 'consumers' of community care: older parents and policy discourse. In M. Caltabiano, R. Hill, R. Frangos (eds) *Achieving Inclusion: Exploring Issues in Disability*. Townsville, Queensland: Centre for Social Welfare Research, James Cook University, pp. 129–146.

Stoel-Gammon, C. (1990) Phonological analysis of four Down's syndrome children. *Applied Psycholinguistics*, **1**, 8–12.

Taylor, S. E., Armor, D. A. (1996) Positive illusions and coping with adversity. *J Pers*, **64**, 873–898.

Thorne, S. (1993) *Negotiating Health Care: The Social Context of Chronic Illness*. Newbury Park CA: Sage.

Tingey, C., Mortensen, L., Matheson, P., Doret, W. (1991) Developmental attainment of infants and young children with Down syndrome. *Int J Disabil Dev Educ*, **38**, 15–26.

Townsend, A., Franks, M. M. (1995) Binding ties: closeness and conflict in adult children's caregiving relationship. *Psychol Aging*, **10**, 342–351.

Van Riper, M. (1999) Maternal perceptions of family-provider relationships and well-being in families of children with Down syndrome. *Research in Nursing and Health*, **22**, 357–368.

Van Riper, M., Pridham, K., Ryff, C. (1992) Symbolic interactionism: a perspective for understanding parent-nurse interactions following the birth of a child with Down syndrome. *Matern Child Nurs J*, **20**, 21–40.

Vondracek, F. W., Skorikov, V. B. (1997) Leisure, school and work activities preferences and their role in vocational identity development. *Career Dev Q*, **45**, 322–340.

Wilgosh, L., Nota, L., Scorgie, K., Soresi, S. (2004) Effective life management in parents of children with disabilities: a cross-national extension. *Dev Disabil Bull*, **26**, 301–312.

Wisniewski, K. E., Kida, E., Albertini, G. (2004) Down syndrome and Alzheimer's disease. In J. A. Rondal, A. Rasore-Quartino, S. Soresi (eds) *The Adult with Down Syndrome. A New Challenge for Society.* London: Whurr, pp. 99–111.

Wood, B. (1993) Planning for the transfer of care: social and psychological issues. In K. Roberto (ed.) *The Elderly Caregiver: Caring for Adults with Developmental Disabilities.* Newbury Park CA: Sage, pp. 95–108.

Zigman, W. B., Seltzer, G. B., Silverman, W. P. (1994) Behavioral and mental health changes associated with aging in adults with mental retardation. In M. M. Seltzer, M. W. Krauss, M. P. Janicki (eds) *Life Course Perspectives on Adulthood and Old Age.* Washington DC: American Association on Mental Retardation, pp. 67–92.

CONCLUSIONS

The specificity question is one of the most difficult to deal with but we are conscious of opening a new perspective on Down syndrome (DS) with this book. For a long time, following the discovery of its aetiology, DS was considered a prototype for moderate and severe mental retardation. Since then, thanks to great progress in molecular genetics, a large number of genetic syndromes conducive to varying degrees of mental retardation have been identified. Some of them have received enough attention to warrant medical, neurophysiological, neurocognitive, psycholinguistic, personality, and/or socioeducational investigation – hence the question of the commonality or specificity of the symptoms documented in the various syndromes.

As the chapters have suggested, the balance is in favour of the existence of syndromic specificity in the behavioural, neurological, medical and personality aspects of DS. The evidence for this comes from intersyndromic comparisons. In particular, there is general agreement that children with DS show a specific developmental profile – strengths in social understanding and as visual learners and difficulties with motor progress, some aspects of language, speech and verbal short-term memory.

Early and later intervention, education, health and psychological care and assistance should be based on this knowledge if they are to be maximally effective. It is essential that people in practice and applied fields know about this and adapt their educational and clinical approaches to the specific needs of people with DS as well as other genetic syndromes associated with mental retardation. It could even be considered that the paradigm that used to be dominant in this field – which assumed that psychometric indications were the most important markers of mental retardation, the aetiological variables being of concern only to the medical profession – has retarded the move towards more efficient therapeutic approaches given its lack of specificity, which favoured poorly focused remedial procedures.

Theoretically, the challenge is of the utmost importance. The behavioural specificity in DS corresponds to particulars uncovered at brain structure level, biochemistry, functions and is related to the DS genotype. Research into genetics and brain function in typically developing individuals is progressing rapidly as we now make use of noninvasive techniques, which are leading to an excellent understanding of how the brain works. As knowledge about

Down Syndrome: Neurobehavioural Specificity. Edited by JA Rondal and J Perera.
© 2006 John Wiley & Sons Ltd.

normal brain function increases we are able to discover more and more about the neurological effects of the extra chromosome 21.

Many problems, of course, are left for further investigation. Our objective was simply to set the stage for more sophisticated research pursuits. Among the steps needed to establish more detailed neurobehavioural profiles and to move forward in the study of the relationships between genes, environment and disorders are deepening interdisciplinary research efforts to go beyond the present state of data juxtaposition into data integration and comprehensive theorising. In particular, we need additional studies that:

- target the genes that contribute to the disorders in different syndromes
- identify environmental factors influencing the developmental projections regarding the phenotypes

We are confident that further work will proceed rapidly on the aspects defined and the questions raised in the present essay. This trend of basic research, rich with theoretical and practical implications, will eventually carry us towards a better understanding of the DS phenotypic realities and their genotypic underpinnings.

Jean-Adolphe Rondal and Juan Perera

Index

Abeta protein
  metabolism of 38
  mitochondrial function affected
    by 45
  overproduction of 36
abortion
  parents' attitudes to 200
  rate 54
accelerated ageing, and Down
    syndrome 10, 36-7
actions, control of 161
acute lymphoblastic leukaemia 56
acute megakaryoblastic leukaemia 56
  pathogenesis 57
  treatment of 58
acute myeloblastic leukaemia 56
adolescents with Down syndrome
  development of personal identity 203
  at end of compulsory schooling 195,
    196, 203
  parents' challenges and tasks 195-6
age-related decline in memory 9, 90, *91*
ageing
  and Down syndrome 8-9, 36-7
  metabolic changes in 37-42
alalia (failure to develop language) 108
Alzheimer's disease (AD)
  characteristic features 45, 93
  metabolic changes in 37-42
  neuropathological signs 36, 93
  susceptibility in Down syndrome
    individuals 8-9, 35-6, 71, 93, 197
amyloid plaques
  major component of 36
  in mouse model 43

amyloid precursor protein (APP)
  encoded by chromosome 21 genes 23,
    35-6
  metabolism of 38
Angelman syndrome
  genetic causes 109
  language profile 109
  prevalence 109
antioxidants
  age-related learning and memory
    losses affected by 43
  see also glutathione
arousal deficits, early intervention
    affected by *181*, 182
articulatory loop
  in working memory 159
  see also auditory phonological loop
associations, Down syndrome support
    10-11
asthma, reduced incidence 10, 60
atlanto-axial instability 56
atrioventricular septal defect 55
attention
  meaning of term 160
  theories of
    Broadbent (filter) model 160
    Norman-Shallice model 160-1
audiological disorders 9, 69, 90
  early intervention affected by 177,
    178
auditory phonological loop, in working
    memory 87, 88-90, 159
auditory short-term memory 74, 88-90
  impairment in Down syndrome 77,
    162, *178*

Down Syndrome: Neurobehavioural Specificity. Edited by JA Rondal and J Perera.
© 2006 John Wiley & Sons Ltd.

542542

This item is to be returned on or before the last due date stamped below .
Items can be renewed 3 times unseen.If a fourth renewal is required the item must be brought to the library.

Liverpool Hope University
The Sheppard-Worlock Library
Tel: 0151 291 2000
http://www.hope.ac.uk/llis